D1082775

Inside Assisted Living

Inside Assisted Living

The Search for Home

J. KEVIN ECKERT
PAULA C. CARDER
LESLIE A. MORGAN
ANN CHRISTINE FRANKOWSKI
ERIN G. ROTH

With contributions by
Sheryl Zimmerman
Lynn Keimig
Robert L. Rubinstein
John G. Schumacher
Debra Dobbs
Tommy B. Piggee, Jr.
and Leanne J. Clark

Foreword by Bill Thomas, M.D.

The Johns Hopkins University Press

Baltimore

© 2009 The Johns Hopkins University Press
All rights reserved. Published 2009
Printed in the United States of America on acid-free paper
9 8 7 6 5 4 3 2 1

The Johns Hopkins University Press
2715 North Charles Street
Baltimore, Maryland 21218-4363
www.press.jhu.edu

Library of Congress Cataloging-in-Publication Data

Inside assisted living : the search for home / J. Kevin Eckert ... [et al.] ; with contributions by
Sheryl Zimmerman ... [et al.] ; foreword by Bill Thomas.
        p. ; cm.
  Includes bibliographical references and index.
  ISBN-13: 978-0-8018-9259-2 (hardcover : alk. paper)
  ISBN-10: 0-8018-9259-7 (hardcover : alk. paper)
  ISBN-13: 978-0-8018-9260-8 (pbk. : alk. paper)
  ISBN-10: 0-8018-9260-0 (pbk. : alk. paper)
   1. Congregate housing—United States. 2. Long-term care facilities—United
States. 3. Patients—United States—Interviews. I. Eckert, J. Kevin.
   [DNLM: 1. Assisted Living Facilities—United States. 2. Patients—United States—
Interview. 3. Homes for the Aged—United States. WT 27 AA1 I59 2009]
  HV1454.2.U6I56 2009
  362.6′10973—dc22   2008037843

A catalog record for this book is available from the British Library.

*Special discounts are available for bulk purchases of this book. For more information, please
contact Special Sales at 410-516-6936 or specialsales@press.jhu.edu.*

The Johns Hopkins University Press uses environmentally friendly book materials, including
recycled text paper that is composed of at least 30 percent post-consumer waste, whenever possible. All of our book papers are acid-free, and our jackets and covers are printed on paper with
recycled content.

Contents

....

Contributors

PAULA C. CARDER, PH.D., assistant professor, Institute on Aging, School of Community Health, Portland State University, Portland, Oregon

LEANNE J. CLARK, M.G.S., PH.D. candidate, graduate research assistant, Center for Aging Studies, The Erickson School, University of Maryland, Baltimore County, Baltimore, Maryland

DEBRA DOBBS, PH.D., assistant professor, School of Aging Studies, University of South Florida, Tampa, Florida

J. KEVIN ECKERT, PH.D., director, Center for Aging Studies at the Erickson School and Department of Sociology and Anthropology, University of Maryland, Baltimore County, Baltimore, Maryland

ANN CHRISTINE FRANKOWSKI, PH.D., senior research associate, Center for Aging Studies, The Erickson School; adjunct assistant professor, Department of Sociology and Anthropology, University of Maryland, Baltimore County, Baltimore, Maryland

LYNN KEIMIG, M.H.A., Ph.D. candidate, ethnographer and project coordinator, Center for Aging Studies, The Erickson School, University of Maryland, Baltimore County, Baltimore, Maryland

LESLIE A. MORGAN, PH.D., professor, Department of Sociology and Anthropology, University of Maryland, Baltimore County, Baltimore, Maryland

TOMMY B. PIGGEE, JR., M.A., CHES, Ph.D. candidate in gerontology, University of Maryland, Baltimore County, Baltimore, Maryland

ERIN G. ROTH, M.A., senior research analyst/ethnographer, Center for Aging Studies, The Erickson School, University of Maryland, Baltimore County, Baltimore, Maryland

ROBERT L. RUBINSTEIN, PH.D., professor, Department of Sociology and Anthropology, University of Maryland, Baltimore County, Baltimore, Maryland

JOHN G. SCHUMACHER, PH.D., associate professor, Department of Sociology and Anthropology; associate director, Center for Aging Studies, The Erickson School, University of Maryland, Baltimore County, Baltimore, Maryland

SHERYL ZIMMERMAN, PH.D., professor and director of aging research, School of Social Work; co-director, UNC Interdisciplinary Center for Aging Research; co-director, Program on Aging, Disability and Long-Term Care, Cecil F. Sheps Center for Health Service Research, University of North Carolina at Chapel Hill, Chapel Hill, North Carolina

Foreword

....

The use of "voice" in the written language has been found as early as 1290, but voices themselves are ancient, as old as humanity itself. Voices are the carriers of culture; they contain our stories, transmit our beliefs, and communicate our emotions. But voices alone are not enough. To influence the wider world, voices must be paired with listeners.

The power of listening pulses between these covers. The act of careful, attentive listening grants this book its scope and power. As I immersed myself in its pages, I was returned to the earliest days of my career in the field of aging. In the early 1990s, I was a young physician and my heart was set on a career in emergency medicine. Then, as so often happens in the field of aging, fate intervened. I was offered a part-time position as the medical director of a small, rural, skilled nursing facility, and I went to work caring for the elders who lived there.

I soon understood that something was terribly wrong. Even though my patients were receiving the best, most up-to-date medical treatment available, they withered and died. They were being fed, clothed, bathed, and entertained, and their care was being delivered in a state-of-the-art facility, but they did not have lives worth living. I pored over my textbooks and journals but found no answers there. Searching for understanding, I began to go to the nursing home when I was off duty. I would sit quietly with a black-and-white speckled composition notebook on my lap. I spent hours there. Listening.

It was there that I first heard the voices of the elders.

I was launched, accidentally, on my career as an amateur ethnographer, filling many notebooks with observations that shaped the course of my career. Fortunately, superbly trained, expert professionals have the capacity to go much deeper, to see more and explain more than I could dream of doing. They plumb the social worlds within which people move, laying bare the behaviors, values, and meanings that define human cultures. This singular capacity forms the core strength of *Inside Assisted Living*. This work does not dabble in easy answers or offer false certainties. Rather, it propels the reader toward new questions and new understandings. Here we explore the balance between minute, everyday details and the social structures that elders and those who care for elders share.

The best example of this virtue is the extended examination of the concept of "aging in place" in these pages. What do these words mean to elders? What does the concept imply to professionals? What do family members think when they hear the words? It turns out that "aging in place" is a complex and densely irregular cultural construct. For some, it is a literal "till death do us part" injunction that requires an elder to remain in his or her own dwelling, no matter what. Others find in the term a more flexible ideal that allows for "home-making" wherever an elder may be living. The authors offer the reader a delightful intellectual voyage.

Home

Heart

Belonging

Welcoming

Community

Celebration

Memory

Connection

and Disconnection

Warmth

Tenderness

Fear

Guilt

Forgiveness

Hope

The field of aging services is being remade, all around us, every day. A system that once required older people to surrender autonomy in exchange for assistance is now finding its way along a new path. We are making a world in which elders can expect that those who come to their aid will adapt their practices, change their attitudes, and alter their structures, schedules, and routines to join with elders as they are.

This is new.

This context allows the voices of our elders to gain new importance. They can lead us, if we will take the time to listen. They can inspire us, if we are willing to be moved by their words. We must listen not so that elders can command our obedience but so that they might lead us to the new questions that we should be asking. Within the deep nature of human elderhood, influence has always been more precious than power.

This book, like all of the best qualitative research, does not aim for "definitive answers" but rather challenges the reader's assumptions with carefully developed personal narratives. Here we find the voices that can take us inside assisted living. Listen as they whisper to us the news of a world waiting to be born.

Bill Thomas, M.D.
Professor of Aging Studies
Erickson School of Aging Studies
University of Maryland, Baltimore County

Preface

··

The goal of this book is to provide readers with an insider's perspective on assisted living through the experiences of those who reside and work there.

Inside Assisted Living is composed of ten chapters and a technical appendix. Chapter 1 sets out the purpose of the book, explains the study design, and discusses the emergence of assisted living as an increasingly popular supportive living alternative for older adults. Chapters 2 through 7 focus on each of six assisted living settings we studied in Maryland, with entry provided through the eyes of a selected resident. Interviews and observations from other individuals within and associated with each provide additional details. This strategy provides a "mini-ethnography" of each place that addresses topics such as how it feels to live in a group setting, the occurrence of age-related changes over time and the employees' responses to those changes, how the setting functions as a business, and firsthand accounts of what it is like to live and work in assisted living. Each of these chapters also points to key findings of our research about the assisted living sector today—including its achievements and challenges.

During the course of this five-year study, we completed 379 ethnographic interviews with residents, their families, and their caregivers in addition to several thousand hours of participant observation in the selected facilities, and attended monthly public meetings on regulatory issues. (More details on how the project was conducted are provided in the Appendix.) The words of the people we spoke to provide a richly detailed story that informs us about the intricate nature of these places.

The following paragraphs provide a brief introduction to the individuals and settings we studied. We developed pseudonyms for each of the assisted living facilities that reflect the culture of each place. Pseudonyms are also used for all persons interviewed. Some of the settings had a casual climate in which everyone was referred to by first name; others were more formal. Our selection of names reflects this. In addition, we altered certain details of both the assisted living settings and the persons interviewed to protect the identities of those involved.

Chapter 2 features Miss Helen at Valley Glen Home, a single-family residence originally converted into a group home for up to eight residents. Miss Helen, disabled by a stroke that left her unable to speak, walk, or assist with any of her own personal care needs, had lived at Valley Glen for two years when we met her, and she was not the only resident with this level of impairment cared for by Rani, the owner-operator.

The next chapter describes Opal, a woman with mild cognitive impairment who finds that living in a small home is the "most boring life you can imagine." Franciscan House, like Valley Glen, is a converted single-family residence licensed as an assisted living facility. Although Opal sometimes wonders if she should have moved into a larger setting with more social activities, she had been a resident for two years when we met her and still lived there at a follow-up three years later.

Karen introduces us to life in Huntington Inn in Chapter 4. Karen had multiple chronic conditions that limited her mobility but not her mind; she was engaged in the daily events at this medium-sized residence and provided insight not only about her own experience, but also about other residents and the employees. Mr. Hill, the owner-operator of Huntington Inn, worked as a nursing home administrator before getting into the assisted living business, and he shares his views on how the industry has changed and will continue to change in the future.

Mrs. Koehler's story in Chapter 5 acquaints us with Middlebury Manor, a family-owned and decidedly middle-class assisted living residence attached to a nursing home. After a dramatic and devastating fall down the stairs in her home, Mrs. Koehler chose Middlebury Manor, in part because of her familiarity with the owners. As the story unfolds, Mrs. Koehler's time there hangs in the balance as her chronic health issues require frequent stays in the hospital and nursing home. Safety, liability, and the desire to "age in place" come into play as the administrators, Mrs. Koehler's daughter, and Mrs. Koehler struggle with these decisions.

Chapter 6 details the story of Dr. Catherine, an educated woman who was well aware of her dementia diagnosis at the time we met her, soon after her daughter insisted that she move into assisted living. The daughter decided on the Chesapeake for its ambiance, cleanliness, reputation, pet policy (her mother had a small dog), and location (near a long-time friend of Dr. Catherine). This chapter provides insight into the processes and decisions involved in making two transitions, an initial one into assisted living and then a second to a separate dementia care unit within the building.

In Chapter 7, Mr. Sidney introduces us to life at Laurel Ridge, a two-level assisted living residence in a heavily trafficked suburban community just outside a large East Coast city. After a hospital stay, Mr. Sidney agreed to enter Laurel Ridge at the prompting of his physician and his late wife's niece, who oversees his care. He holds a balanced view of life in his new home, appreciating having someone to manage his medications, regular meals, and people to talk with, while showing surprise at the frailty and discordant behavior of other residents and disdain for management decisions.

The final three chapters draw on our findings from all six facilities and many residents' stories to address some cross-cutting themes. Chapter 8 describes everyday life in assisted living, focusing primarily on the residents' perspective. The next chapter focuses on stability and change over time, including the critical aging-in-place philosophy and whether it is realized in assisted living facilities. Chapter 10 focuses on eight core realities of assisted living today as well as promises and challenges for the future. A technical appendix provides a detailed description of the research design and methods used in the ethnographic study.

As we launch into our exploration of life inside assisted living, we thank the residents, families, and staff members who willingly spoke with us over the course of the study. Without their time and interest, there would be no story to tell. We also thank the National Institute on Aging (NIA), one of the National Institutes of Health, for providing the funding that enabled us to conduct the study "Transitions in Assisted Living: Socio-cultural Aspects" (RO1 AG019345). We hope that our readers will find this book helpful in understanding assisted living as it exists today.

Inside Assisted Living

ONE

❀❦ Introduction

You know, that was my impression—that this is the last place. And I see these people lined up in wheelchairs in these homes. And I thought, well, there they sit, just waiting to die. So that was my idea of it.

And then when my son thought that I had to make a change, I thought, well, I'll try it. He brought me over here and we looked at it and I just, you know, came along with it. I wasn't enthusiastic, but I just came along with it. And I made up my mind that I was here for a reason. So I tried to look at all the good parts. And I just settled in until it's become my home. And I'm very, very happy here.

The best thing about living here is that I don't have to cook. I don't miss anything. I feel like, if I was in my apartment [before moving into assisted living], I'm alone, you know, and I have to go out looking for excitement or doing things. Here I can choose.

—RESIDENT OF THE CHESAPEAKE ASSISTED LIVING

Some of us are familiar with long-term care and with assisted living as a long-term care option. But for a lot of people, questions and concerns are many. For instance, what choices do older people have when they require daily assistance to cook, dress, bathe, or take medications? Who monitors their chronic medical conditions and/or protects them from risks associated with cognitive impairment? How do we as a society respond to older persons who can no longer live independently in the community, but don't need (or want) to move into a nursing facility? Increasingly, the answer to these questions is "assisted living."

The purpose of this book is to introduce readers to life in assisted living from the perspectives of individuals who reside or work in one of six actual settings in Maryland. We believe that this type of supportive housing cannot be fully understood unless we go inside different assisted living residences to learn about day-to-day life directly from those who live or work there. By telling their stories and relating those stories to the larger arena of long-term care, we examine some key dilemmas facing those who live in, work in, and regulate such settings. Moreover, learning more about assisted living benefits all of us as we think about the alternatives available to our families and our future selves.

Over the past decade, the question of what assisted living is, should be, or should not be has consumed the time of many gerontologists and long-term care experts. These individuals have weighed in on this question as they work to develop sensible regulations and engage in influential research. Still, at both the state and the national levels, people express uncertainty and dissatisfaction, as well as varying levels of optimism, when discussing assisted living. In this book, we let the real experts—residents, their families, and employees—tell about assisted living in their own words.

How these people experience life and work inside assisted living is important, because their stories educate those of us who are or will someday be considering such a move for ourselves or a family member. But beyond that, their stories serve to inform current practice and policy-making by providing a more complete understanding of what assisted living currently is and how we would like it to be. Assisted living facilities are complex places, made so by the intersection of individual lives, political and economic factors, social and cultural beliefs, and conflicting expectations.

When we set out to study the nature of daily life inside six diverse settings, we did not directly ask older persons to define "assisted living." Instead, we let them tell us their stories: how and why they came to live in an assisted living residence; what they do on a daily basis; about their neighbors, friends, and enemies, as well as the employees they preferred and the ones to avoid; and their opinions about the many spoken and unspoken rules and restrictions. They also shared their fears and disappointments as well as surprise at how nice some settings could be compared with the negative image of a nursing home so many had held in their minds.

Within the six settings we studied are residents, their engaged family members, and the staff, who are collectively active in composing the mundane and exceptional events that constitute the reality of daily life. By talking to these groups and observing their interactions and routines, we present an authentic view of how life in assisted living unfolds in all its complexity and diversity.

Over the past decade, assisted living has become one of the most popular and familiar alternatives for care of older adults who need daily assistance or supervision or who find it difficult to manage in their own homes. Its popularity is demonstrated by the expanding numbers of residents and settings (Mollica, Johnson-Lamarche, and O'Keeffe 2005) as well as growing state interest in regulation (Bruce 2006; Carlson 2005). In the media, assisted living is variously portrayed as a retirement option for wealthy persons who need only minimal support services, as a business that reduces seniors to poverty before unceremoniously discharging them to nursing facilities, or as the new (but unregulated) addition to the nursing home scene.

For example, an investigation by *Consumer Reports* revealed that "finding a good, safe, and affordable facility has . . . become problematic for seniors and their families. There's a lot to consider: the setting, the cost, the array of services, the condition of the other residents, the solvency of the company, not to mention the rights of residents to stay, or the necessity for them to go, if their condition deteriorates." The report especially criticized the "hodgepodge" of state regulations that result in a wide range of settings that fall under the label "assisted living" (Consumer Reports 2005). A more recent CBS Evening News report focused on the negative aspects and called for more stringent regulations that impose sanctions and accountability for poor care (CBS Evening News 2006).

But assisted living has also been presented in a more positive light, as the following suggests: "Reinvent the nursing home and the result might look a lot like assisted living. Instead of the shared rooms of a nursing home, residents live in private apartments, usually with kitchenettes and bathrooms. There's staff available to help residents eat, bathe, and dress" (Shapiro 2001). In practice, assisted living can be any or all of the above.

While there are varying formal definitions, in practice assisted living is the large middle ground between receiving care at home, often with the assistance of family and/or professionals, and admission to a nursing home, a setting of last resort according to most public surveys. Often older persons move into an assisted living residence as an alternative to home care that doesn't provide enough support (e.g., does not have the ability to respond to unscheduled needs) or as an alternative to a nursing facility that, for lack of a better description, provides too much support (e.g., provides assistance in bathing or taking medications whether the individual requires help or not). Home health care is defined as care "provided in the place of residence for the purpose of promoting, maintaining, or restoring health in maximizing the level of independence while minimizing the effects of disability and illness, including terminal illness" (NCHS 2007). Services provided in home health care can include skilled nursing care, the availability of special-needs equipment, administration of medications, and personal, hospice, and psychosocial care. The same set of services might also be provided in nursing facilities and assisted living residences, though states place limits on the level of services assisted living may provide; for example, ongoing skilled nursing care cannot be provided. Nationally, more people needing care reside in nursing homes (1.6 million), with 1.4 million receiving home care (NCHS 2007) and about 1 million in assisted living facilities (NCAL 2007). It is worth noting that the number of nursing home residents has remained stable over the past 20 years in spite of the increasing population of older persons (Redfoot 2005). Of course, assisted living cannot take full credit for this decline in the use of nursing facilities, but its growth has been and continues to be a major factor.[1]

During our research, residents and their families, when describing their need for long-term care services, frequently discussed their desire for something other than a nursing facility. For example, the son of one assisted living resident we interviewed said: "When my grandparents were in a nursing home, I wouldn't go. I went a couple of times and I couldn't stand . . . the smell." We heard similar accounts from other family members and residents, some of whom had not been in a nursing home for many years. Similarly, the assisted living administrators and employees we interviewed often defined assisted living by comparing it with a nursing home, explaining that the former was preferable to the latter. Of course, nursing home operators and advocates might rightly take issue with this comparison; the point here is that many people perceive nursing homes to be an undesirable form of long-term care.

In fact, assisted living as a distinct type of senior housing is, in large part, the result of three individuals' dissatisfaction with nursing homes. Stimulated by long-term care experiences in their own families, Keren Brown Wilson in Oregon and Paul and Teresa Klaassen in Virginia each adopted philosophical principles for housing with services distinctly in contrast to those of nursing homes and in-home nursing services (Wilson 2007). These principles, developed in the 1980s, included respect for resident independence, choice, and privacy in an apartment-style building designed to be "homelike" and noninstitutional. The regulatory responses of the two states differed. Oregon allowed assisted living providers to deliver a level of service comparable to what used to be called "intermediate" care in nursing homes; that is, assisted living could provide all but ongoing 24-hour skilled nursing care. Affordability for low- to moderate-income persons was a central tenet of the initial demonstration in that state.[2] In the 1990s, some Oregon policymakers and providers argued that the promise of assisted living should be to "age in place," by which they meant that an individual should be able to remain in the assisted living residence as long as the person's medical condition did not require full-time skilled nursing care.

In contrast, Virginia developed fairly restrictive criteria regarding the degree of physical or cognitive impairment acceptable for newly admitted assisted living residents, but that state's regulations allowed residents to arrange third-party services beyond meals, housekeeping, and basic assistance with activities of daily living. Thus, remaining in the assisted living facility as health and functioning changed was possible but depended on the resident's ability to locate and pay for the necessary additional services, as well as the management's willingness to retain people who needed more care.

While Oregon and Virginia might get the credit for jump-starting the growth of an assisted living industry, throughout the 1990s other states and private companies quickly followed their lead. The popular definition to emerge during this time asserted that assisted living settings operate under a "social model" of care, including a homelike living environment, with respect for residents' privacy, choices, independence, dignity, and individuality (Wilson 1990; Kane and Wilson 2001). While perhaps challenging to realize in practice, these social model principles, developed in contrast to the medical model of the nursing home, were integral to the emergence and growth of assisted living. From the beginning, Oregon's regulations defined assisted living in contrast to its long-term care sister, the nursing home, as text from a 1989 state policy paper indicates: "We are developing educational modules [to explain] how the social model is different from the medical model. Assisted Living demonstrates this difference in physical structure and support services for the residents. The outcome of the residents is better: they have more independence, more choices in living, more dignity, and they live in a homelike environment that continuously treats them with respect and keeps their privacy in mind" (SDSD 1989, 5).

That Oregon policy paper goes on to explain that the social model is enacted via the "physical structure" by providing private apartments with bathrooms, kitchenettes, locking doors, and individual temperature controls.[3] Support services were to be individualized, based on each resident's personal needs and preferences. For example, a resident should have a choice of whether or not to accept employee assistance to take a shower, and residents would be permitted to direct their own care.

A more recent study of Oregon's assisted living program describes the various efforts that policymakers and operators made to establish this new form of long-term care as distinct from nursing homes (Carder 2002a). The phrase "social model" was consistently attributed to assisted living by policymakers, while "medical model" was used to describe nursing homes and hospitals. For example, the social model would address a resident's medical diagnosis as only one of several needs, with similar importance given to the individual's psychosocial needs, personal preferences, and financial needs. In contrast, the medical model focuses primarily on the person's medical diagnosis and treatment. Oregon's assisted living regulations in particular defined six philosophical elements of the social model: a homelike environment and support of residents' independence, privacy, dignity, individuality, and choice. Assisted living operators also employ a new vocabulary; they intentionally refer to *resident* (instead of *patient*), *apartment* (instead of *room* or *bed*), and *residence* or *community* (instead of *facility*) to distinguish themselves from nursing homes (Carder 2002a, 2002b). Today, most states use some version of the social model in their regulatory definition (Mollica, Johnson-Lamarche, and O'Keeffe 2005), although the extent to which this philosophy is realized in practice remains an open question.

In addition to the social model, many providers and advocates identified "aging in place" as both a goal and a probable outcome of the new assisted living sector. The phrase was used by demographers to describe the finding, confirmed by surveys and geographic data (Prisuta, Barrett, and Evans 2006) that older persons desired to age where they have lived; they preferred not to move, especially to a nursing home. Thus, a move into assisted living might be the last move an older person would make. Although Oregon regulations did not define aging in place, it continues to be a hot topic both there and in national policy discussions. We return to this topic in Chapter 9.

Another key issue in this research and also nationally concerns the economics of assisted living. Cost issues affect the older persons and their families who are paying for services, as well as assisted living operators. By and large, assisted living caters to a private-pay market. Forty-one states now use public resources to subsidize the cost of assisted living services (Mollica, Johnson-Lamarche, and O'Keeffe 2005), but these subsidies are available only to low-income individuals who need nursing-home-level care. In addition, states limit the number of subsidies available, the scope of services, and reimbursement amounts to providers, resulting in a gap between demand and availability (Justice and Heestand 2003; O'Keeffe and Wiener 2004). Projections show that the need for affordable assisted living will increase significantly with the aging of the population (Golant 2005/06).

Many assisted living providers are hesitant to accept publicly subsidized clients because reimbursement rates do not cover their operational costs. The expenses of operating a facility, including liability insurance, employee salaries and benefits, building maintenance, and the record-keeping demanded by regulations, are often mentioned by assisted living owner-operators as reasons for accepting only those who have the resources to pay privately. However, not all operators can choose to accept only private-pay residents; they would rather have a subsidized client paying a lower rate than an empty unit.

Early in its development, assisted living was viewed by many as a remedy for the concerns that people expressed about nursing homes, especially the institutional- and hospital-like environment and the lack of privacy, dignity, and independence afforded to people living there. For example, in 1993 Donna Shalala, then secretary of Health and Human Services, wrote that "assisted living is an example of the good news in aging. States, local governments, private corporations, and the frail elderly themselves, have creatively met the need for care at reasonable cost while maintaining the individual's dignity and independence" (Shalala 1993).

During the initial period of assisted living growth (the 1980s into the 1990s), some states struggled to keep up with the private industry's momentum to develop more residences. Nursing home apologists argued that assisted living was an "end run" around the stringent regulations to which nursing homes were held accountable. Topics of debate then, as now, included whether to require licensed nurses in assisted living facilities, whether and how to define and monitor this new form of long-term care, whether and at what level to set staffing ratios, and what range of medical services would be permitted. During this time, national trade and professional groups formed to advocate for the social model, or at least to prevent a medical model to define, regulate, and monitor the new assisted living type of housing and care.

Many states reorganized their existing residential care programs under the heading of "assisted living," including board-and-care and group homes that housed anywhere from two to more than one hundred persons. Other states reserved the "assisted living" title for the new settings specifically built for this purpose. The decision to combine a wide range of diverse settings and programs under a single label confused the public as well as investors, government agencies, and senior housing operators. Advocates and policymakers remain divided on whether a national definition and regulatory framework, rather than the current state-based approach, should be implemented.

The honeymoon period for assisted living was short lived, as reports of substandard care and consumers' unmet expectations quickly attracted media attention. Studies conducted in the mid- to late 1990s revealed a lack of clarity regarding the definition and boundaries of assisted living (Hawes et al. 1995), a problem that persists today as states, advocates, and providers debate what it is or should be (ALW 2003; Carlson 2005; Kane and Wilson 2001). Over time, the idea of aging in place came into question, as residents with growing needs for personal care or medical services were moved out of assisted living homes and into nursing homes or residential care settings. A public report criticized the adequacy of state licensure to protect consumers (GAO 1999). Wilson noted that "in less than ten years assisted living had gone from poster child to long-term care's bad boy" (2007).

Although proponents of assisted living originally set out to distinguish this new sector from nursing homes, today it is sometimes described as "a nursing home in denial" or as "the nursing home of twenty years ago." Increasingly these descriptions may be appropriate as the number and severity of physical and cognitive limitations among residents increase over time (Golant 2008). Recent studies indicate that a large percentage of assisted living residents have some form or level of cognitive impairment (Rosenblatt et al. 2004; Morgan, Gruber-Baldini, and Magaziner 2001; Zimmerman et al. 2005a). Although we discuss these issues in more detail in the following chapters, a brief review of historical threads provides a background and a framework for understanding assisted living as it exists today.

How New Is the Concept of Assisted Living?

Is assisted living truly a "new" alternative, or is it simply a spin on an old standard? Assisted living developed from a wide range of social and cultural forces, not the least of which was consumer dissatisfaction with nursing homes. While the contemporary nursing home is a relative newcomer to U.S. society, communities have always needed to provide for individuals or groups not able to live independently. Throughout history, individuals who lacked either personal or financial resources relied on a patchwork of local charitable organizations. For individuals without family or strong ties to an ethnic or religious group, the only alternative was the public poorhouse or a religious or service organization almshouse.

After the enactment of Social Security in 1935, "a whole new era in entrepreneurial ventures sprang forth. Privately operated rest homes and nursing homes and convalescent homes popped up like ants at a picnic" (Zinn 1999, 31). Newly organized boarding homes, convalescence centers, and hospitals proliferated across the country with little homogeneity among facilities in terms of the services provided or their quality. These unlicensed and unregulated settings were owned and operated by religious, fraternal, or local organizations (Levey and Amidon 1967; Morgan, Eckert, and Lyon 1995; Sherman and Newman 1988). By 1949, only eight states had licensure laws governing medical care facilities and some exempt, publicly run homes (Kinnaman 1949, quoted in Zinn 1999). Even where statutes existed, resources were not available to enforce them, a situation that persists in some states to this day.

In 1952 an interesting and still relevant report by the National Committee on Aging highlighted both the importance of protecting older persons' autonomy and the public confusion regarding the range of senior housing types and services offered. For example, the report authors stated that older people "have the same essential rights and requirements which all people possess: the right to maximum self-determination, privacy of person and thought, and personal dignity." The authors added that "if a resident is to be helped to function to the full extent of his capabilities, he should be free to leave and return at reasonable hours. . . . Residents should be allowed to undertake those normal risks of life which do not involve special dangers to them" (cited in Zinn 1999). The report further criticized the institutional characteristics of long hallways and dormitory-style living typical in long-term care of the early 1900s. These issues are as topical today, with some contemporary settings designed by architects who specialize in buildings that are safe, accessible to people with disabilities, and consumer-oriented (AIA 2007; Regnier 1997).[4]

Federal construction loan programs in the 1950s and the passage of Medicare and Medicaid legislation in 1965 spurred the growth of nursing homes. The number of profit-making nursing home chains increased, and today, the majority of nursing homes are proprietary (Starr 1982, 429). They are also highly regulated and monitored. Federal legislation adopted in 1987[5] brought additional oversight to the long-term care sector, including inspection and enforcement of rules credited with improving the quality of life of nursing home residents.

Despite all of this growth and attention, neither residents nor their families were satisfied with nursing homes as places to live, as indicated by surveys of older persons (Yankelovich 1990) and by the publications and exposés about poor nursing home quality (Mendelson 1974; Sarton 1982; Vladeck 1980). It is noteworthy that assisted living facilities emerged as a nursing home alternative during this point in history. Perhaps assisted living was an idea whose time had come.

Assisted Living Today

Contemporary descriptions of assisted living pick up on themes and aspirations of long-term care advocates and policymakers that date to the early twentieth century, including fostering independence, privacy, dignity, and noninstitutional environments. These concepts thus represent an evolution rather than revolutionary step forward. Yet the label "assisted living" is on its way to replacing other similar terms applied to residential housing for older persons (e.g., "board-and-care," "residential care"). Forty-one states and the District of Columbia use the term "assisted living" as a licensure category (Mollica, Johnson-Lamarche, and O'Keeffe 2005), and most recently a federal workgroup was formed in response to congressional concern about assisted living practices and regulations (ALW 2003). The workgroup included representatives from 48 national organizations, such as consumer advocates, health care professionals, and senior housing providers. How to define assisted living became a major point of disagreement among the workgroup participants, with some insisting that assisted living had to provide private units (as in Oregon) and others demanding that states establish at least two levels of care. Although these issues were not resolved, the following definition was proposed:

> Assisted living is a state regulated and monitored residential long-term care option. Assisted living provides or coordinates oversight and services to meet the residents' individualized scheduled needs, based on the residents' assessment and service plans and their unscheduled needs as they arise. . . . A resident has the right to make choices and receive services in a way that will promote the resident's dignity, autonomy, independence, and quality of life. . . . Assisted living does not generally provide ongoing, 24-hour skilled nursing. (ALW 2003, 12)

The preceding section of this chapter provides a brief overview of definitions of long-term care and the history of assisted living. But what is it like for those who live and work there? In this book, we answer that question.

The Study Approach

To study the everyday life of people who live and work in assisted living, we used an approach called ethnography, a research technique familiar to many social scientists, especially cultural anthropologists. The term is based on the words *ethno*, meaning "people," and *graphy*, referring to the writing about a specific subject or object. This method is designed to collect and interpret cultural information about a group of people in a specific place and time. Since the 1800s there have been many ethnographic studies of small towns and urban neighborhoods, native tribes, schools, occupational groups, and many other communities or settings where people gather to live, work, worship, play, and raise their families.

The "doing" of ethnography involves researchers systematically spending time talking to the people who live or work in a specific place, writing "field notes" that describe what they see, hear and experience, audiotaping interviews, taking photographs, and carefully documenting patterns and unique events of everyday life in a particular place. Field ethnographers (the term we use to describe the researchers who work "in the field") focus on how the members of a place (e.g., family members, workers, students, and teachers) organize, communicate, celebrate, resolve conflicts, and go about their daily lives. These are the elements of culture—the way people do things and the reasons they do them. As researchers, ethnographers want to hear about (through in-depth interviews) and witness (through observation of daily activities) the explanations that people give for how and why things are the way they are in a given place.

The purpose of this study was to understand the types of and reasons for transitions in the lives of current assisted living residents. To conduct ethnography in this setting means spending time in a place that some individuals think of as home and others think of as work. People on both the inside and the outside have definitions of what this place is or should be. State and local government agency personnel, who are responsible for licensing and monitoring assisted living facilities, think of it as a health care setting that must meet written standards of care. Residents and their families are concerned with both care and creating a sense of "home." For this study, we focus primarily on the people who live in the assisted living residence. But we also interviewed family members of older adults; assisted living owners, operators, and staff; government employees who oversee assisted living residences; physicians and hospice personnel working with people living there; volunteers; and members of trade organizations that represent the industry.

Data collection began in the spring of 2002 and continued through the winter of 2007, and included weekly visits over 10-month (on average) consecutive periods at each of the six sites and interviews with more than 300 individuals. While spending time in each setting, our field ethnographers took extensive notes, some of which appear in subsequent chapters, describing the events they saw and heard about. These include routine happenings like meals, informal gatherings of residents, visits from friends and families, scheduled social activities, and the arrival and departure of residents and employees. We also observed events that did not occur on a routine basis such as medical emergencies, regulatory inspections, and building renovation and remodeling.

Over time, the "participant observation" by the field ethnographers included taking part in activities as varied as setting the dining room table, playing the piano in the central living room space, making cookies for a Christmas celebration, and playing checkers, bingo, and other games. When a resident we had interviewed was transferred to a hospital or nursing home, we went to visit. Through spending significant time with our interviewees and participating in these everyday events, we found that our presence became normal and ordinary, permitting access to an "insider's" view of daily life. This ethnographic study reveals the variation within and across these six settings and provides important lessons about aging, managing chronic illness, public policy, social relationships, good-quality care, community, and long-term-care finance. The local culture of each place, its daily routines, joys and sorrows, mix-ups, heroics, the caring, and the jokes—all become real.

We came to see unexpected patterns and to recognize and value the distinctiveness of the individuals who are often simply labeled as "residents" in national discussions of the assisted living setting. Each of these older adults brought to their time in assisted living a distinctive history and background of events, choices, and accomplishments that far exceeded the constellation of health or cognitive issues that led them there. Likewise, the human aspect of these settings was constantly evident as we observed the staff going about their daily tasks and as administrators set the tone for service delivery, addressed changing needs, and negotiated with families, physicians, and social programs on behalf of residents, many of whom were too sick, confused, or overwhelmed to do so on their own behalf.

While we might suspect that assisted living residences providing poorer care would not consent to participate in our study, there were nonetheless clear variations in how well the six we observed met the standards proposed as appropriate both by law and in the literature. Though this study did not focus on "quality of care," we did not see or hear about any instances of abuse, neglect, or mistreatment. Given that spectacular scandals in assisted living and other long-term care settings are the stories most likely to appear in the national press, we are pleased to have the opportunity to represent the efforts of many dedicated men and women who provide daily assistance, in the form of meals, medication administration, hugs, showers, transportation, and clean toilets, to frail older persons, some of whom are not capable of saying "thank you" in words.

TWO

❊❧ Miss Helen at Valley Glen Home

The story of Miss Helen's move to Valley Glen Home begins more than 20 years ago. When asked how her mother came from Tennessee to reside in a small assisted living home in Maryland, Miss Helen's daughter, Alicia, said, "Well, I guess we can almost go back another generation. My grandmother also had Alzheimer's. . . . She lived with us growing up, . . . but at some point in time, she had to enter a nursing home."

In this chapter, we hear a daughter's account of choosing a long-term care setting for her mother. We learn about the importance of the relationship between care provider and care receiver during the settling-in process, and how they work together making operational decisions about who can stay and who must go. The key issues presented in this chapter include the challenges that families face in locating a long-term care setting for a relative; the range of individuals and groups that can be involved in one person's move to an assisted living facility; the importance of the assisted living operator in shaping the local culture; how the individual's needs are defined and determined in conflicting ways by different individuals and groups; and the challenges of finding (or creating) the right fit between person and place.

Introducing Miss Helen

Five older women lived at Valley Glen Home when our research began in the spring of 2002. We chose to focus on Miss Helen because we felt that her unique characteristics and story best exemplify the essence of this small assisted living residence. Miss Helen did not match up to the national statistics on the average assisted living resident because she lacked the ability to talk, feed herself, walk, transfer, or manage any form of personal care without assistance from one—and sometimes two—other people. At 79 years old, she was about five years younger than the national average, and when we met her, she had lived at Valley Glen for a little more than three years, more than the national average of 28 months (NCAL 2007). She would reside there for nearly three more years until her death. Finally, she was the only African American resident at Valley Glen; the other residents were white. Beyond these demographic reasons for focusing on Miss Helen, another motivation for profiling her story came from a compelling description written by the ethnographer who did most of the fieldwork at this setting:

> We were all admiring Miss Helen's marvelous hair, fine elegant braids all over her head. It was beautiful. . . . One of the temporary caregivers, an African woman, took special care to attend to Miss Helen's hair . . . [with] intricate braiding. I marveled at how expressive Miss Helen could be without the ability to lift her head, to voluntarily move much of her body, or to speak. . . . We all commented on it, and it was easy to see Miss Helen responding with delight, even though her range of expressiveness is severely limited. As Matilda [a direct care aide] has indicated, you can tell how she feels. You can tell.

This description is noteworthy: here was an assisted living resident who could not voluntarily move her body and thus required total assistance to do anything. But in this depiction of hair braiding, something much more than "grooming" (to use the standard long-term-care language to describe hair care) was clearly taking place. It was some quality that we did not yet know how to label, yet it was recognizable here and in other examples we observed over time at Valley Glen. Miss Helen's case, we believed, could teach us lessons about the needs of impaired older persons and the capacity of both the individuals and the systems intended to care for them.

Researchers have described the increasing number and severity of health conditions—both physical and cognitive or mental—of assisted living residents in recent years (NCAL 2007; Rosenblatt et al. 2004; Zimmerman et al. 2005a). Miss Helen seemed to represent that trend, if at an extreme level. One component of this study included performance-based evaluation of physical and mental abilities on the "focal case" residents in the study, including evaluation of each individual's concentration and memory, balance, walking speed, muscle strength, and height and weight. The clinical researcher who conducted these assessments used a lengthy set of closed-ended questions and performance-based observations (e.g., ability to rise from a chair and time to walk several feet), and he audio-tape-recorded a clinically focused description of his observation of each resident. During his first meeting with Miss Helen, he recorded this note:

> Miss Helen is sitting in a wheelchair. Her posture/sitting position is such that her chin is nearly touching the left side of her upper chest. Placing myself in a kneeling position, I can see that her eyes are open. Several attempts were made to elicit a response from Miss Helen. Each attempt failed. Miss Helen's cognitive status renders her nonassessable . . . at this time. I will attempt to evaluate her on a later date.

Because Miss Helen could not speak, Rani, the home's owner-operator, provided details to the interviewer, confirming that Miss Helen was totally dependent in all "activities of daily living." How did Rani and her small group of female employees take care of not only Miss Helen, but also Nellie (a resident we describe in more detail below), both of whom required assistance in every aspect of daily life? For how long would they be able to care for two women, along with three others, with this level of impairment? And what was the nature of the care they provided to Miss Helen and the other residents? We tell Miss Helen's story as a way of setting the context for this discussion of the nature of life inside a small assisted living home.

Miss Helen's Move to Valley Glen Home

Miss Helen's daughter, Alicia, provided the details on her mother's life, including events in the months before she came to Valley Glen Home. The story is one of gradual but continual decline, until Alicia accepted that her mother needed to live where she could be supervised so that she did not injure herself or forget to eat, take medications, or do any of the other daily tasks required to continue living in her own home. Her decline follows a typical pattern leading to a move into assisted living.

Miss Helen had been widowed a few years before Alicia's decision to seek assisted living care. She had continued to drive her car and to work as a hairdresser, but Alicia explained that the "subtle signs" of her mother's decline became increasingly obvious. Miss Helen's sisters and friends called Alicia to tell her that her mother was failing and provide detailed examples of her forgetfulness. During that period, Miss Helen voluntarily stopped driving and began attending an adult day center, acknowledging a decline in her health and independence.

Alicia drove to Tennessee each month to check on her mother and began looking into senior housing near her mother's home. With a full-time job and two teenaged sons, Alicia worried that she would not be able to continue visiting on a regular basis, and she faced up to a common family problem—how to participate in and oversee care of a parent at a distance. In addition, Alicia learned that small group homes were not available near her mother's home, and she believed that her mother would not be able to manage in a large facility.

Finally, after an episode when Miss Helen left the stove burner on unattended, it became clear that it was time for her to move. But where? All Alicia knew for certain was that she did not want to place her mother in a nursing home. She recalled that when Miss Helen had placed her own mother in a nursing home, it had "weighed heavily" on her. Alicia now felt renewed sympathy with what her mother had experienced in trying to do the best thing for her parent. In Miss Helen's time, a nursing home was the only available option. Alicia's choices were somewhat broader.

Eventually Alicia moved Miss Helen into her own home for a few weeks as she considered the options, including having her live with the family. During this time, she realized that her mother required more care than she could provide: Alicia's work and family commitments meant that her mother would be left alone for hours at a time in a house that was neither safe nor disabled-accessible. Alicia continued her search.

According to interviews, Alicia's exploration of long-term care settings was guided by personal, professional, and spiritual considerations. She preferred a small, homelike residence for her mother. She hired a private (fee-for-service) case manager to narrow the scope of places she should visit, and she contacted a local Alzheimer's support group, where someone confirmed her instinct that a small setting would be best for someone with dementia. Alicia scanned the long list of licensed assisted living facilities provided by a local county department of aging and called some of them, but it was difficult to appreciate the differences without visiting each one. The private case manager highly recommended Valley Glen Home, so Alicia called and spoke to Rani. Although her search clearly involved legwork, professional input, and money, Alicia also described a spiritual element when she explained that she found Valley Glen "by the grace of God."

She described her first visit to Valley Glen: "It was just a feeling of you are at home . . . just the way the bedrooms are, the decorations, and the . . . it was just a feeling of home." The fact that Rani lived there with her own mother and son added to this feeling. At that time, another African American woman lived at Valley Glen, and Alicia asked Rani if she could call this woman's daughter for a reference. She was relieved after talking to this woman because, as she said, "there is also a stigma . . . in terms of, well, a lot of blacks don't like the concept of not having . . . you are putting your mother away." Talking with a peer who had been through a similar situation confirmed for Alicia that she was making the right decision. Valley Glen Home felt right to Alicia because, as she explained, "I did not want to put her into a nursing home until it was just absolutely necessary, so this was kind of also an in-between thing in terms of just me dealing with the point that I am having to put her anywhere. I can always say, 'Well, no, Mom, I didn't put you in a nursing home.'"

Changing Health

During interviews, Alicia and Rani each independently recalled that when Miss Helen moved into Valley Glen Home she was capable of walking and eating independently, though she was limited in other daily activities, such as bathing and toileting, and did not communicate more than a few words. Alicia signed her mother up for two sessions of adult day care each week as recommended by an Alzheimer's support group, but Miss Helen continued to decline both cognitively and physically. The first change came when Miss Helen stopped feeding herself. Rani attributed this decline to the fact that the staff at the adult day center hand-fed Miss Helen because it took too long for her to feed herself and they needed to keep to a schedule. The second change was more abrupt, as Rani explained: "And then I think she had a small stroke. One night she just fell off her bed. . . . One night she just rolled down and then her neck just started to go off to one side. So they took her to the doctor and to the orthopedic and they had CAT scans . . . and all the things they did and the doctor said, 'There is nothing wrong with her. She just feels comfortable keeping her neck that way.' And then the physician said that she may also have had a stroke."

Alicia also said: "I guess officially on my mother's medical records, . . . it indicates severe dementia. Although the doctors say, yes, it is probably Alzheimer's, but we never went the extra . . . at that point, why pay for extra testing to say, okay, it is officially Alzheimer's?"

To Rani and Alicia, Miss Helen's actual diagnosis was beside the point when it came to meeting her daily needs. We will provide more details about Valley Glen Home and the people who live and work there before returning to Miss Helen's case for additional lessons about long-term care.

Getting to Know Valley Glen Home

Valley Glen Home is located in a quiet residential neighborhood a few blocks off a busy thoroughfare. This pleasant, leafy suburb appeared to be exclusively single-family dwellings with lots of up to one-half acre and with most homes built sometime in the late 1940s or early 1950s. Architectural styles included ranchers, Cape Cods, and colonials. The neighborhood had well-manicured curbs, little or no street parking, no sidewalks, and seasonal displays of spring flowers, flowering shrubs, and large shade trees.

No exterior signs indicated that Valley Glen Home was a licensed care facility. The wheelchair ramp that provided access to the back door and outdoor deck was located toward the back of the long driveway, where it was not visible from the street. There was a basketball hoop at the end of the driveway for Rani's son, a sign that this home was much like any other suburban residence.

The first impression of the interior is captured in an ethnographer's note:

Just inside the front door was the living room . . . no lobby, no receptionist, no neutral territory for greetings, impression management, or segregation of residents from visitors. Once in, we became involved. One woman sat alone in the long, spacious living room that was furnished with clean and otherwise unremarkable furniture. This was the furniture of a discount store: functional, neutral colors, and not designed with disabilities in mind. The furnishings, placed around the walls of the room, created a long open space with a TV at one end. Probably one could view the TV from any seat in this room, the largest common area for residents and their families to gather.

Valley Glen Home was licensed for up to eight residents and at the highest level of care (level 3, described further in the Appendix) permitted by the state rules, in addition to being certified to participate in the state's Medicaid waiver program for assisted living. Typical suburban bedrooms were converted into single or double rooms, some with a curtain to separate sleeping spaces and provide minimal privacy. A few residents brought a favorite chair or a small table, and nearly all had photos or other items to reflect memories and past events. Relatively little other personalization of space was visible. The décor consisted of cheery floral bedspreads and curtains. All meals were shared in a large kitchen/dining room, where Rani cooked and served the meals with the assistance of one employee. A large, family-style dining table with a plastic tablecloth served for most meals. One slightly combative resident, Iveris, received meals separately to minimize stress at the table. A room behind the dining area, containing a sofa where a live-in care provider sometimes slept, led to the other residents' rooms. One of these rooms was occupied by Rani's mother, who, while not a paying customer, was no less a recipient of services at Valley Glen Home. Although not officially a dementia care facility, Valley Glen did house mostly residents with dementia; some had other physical ailments as well.

Rani's Story

Before immigrating to the United States, Rani had lived in India with her husband and son; her sister, Priya, had lived in the United States for more than 20 years. After their father died, Priya encouraged Rani and their mother to come to Maryland. In India, Rani had completed a master's degree in psychology and begun a Ph.D. in management, but she abandoned her studies to care for several elderly relatives, including her father, her in-laws, and an uncle. Rani's husband remained in India with the plan of moving to Maryland at some point. But after Rani and her husband had lived seven years in separate countries, he died in India before his immigration paperwork was completed.

Priya researched the costs, benefits, and rules related to operating a group home and suggested that it would be a good way for Rani to earn a living in the United States and care for their 85-year-old mother as well as Rani's teenaged son. The two sisters were co-owners of Valley Glen Home, but Rani lived there and provided the daily care for residents with the assistance of hired staff. Priya, who lived in a neighboring county and worked full time at an office job, took care of administrative duties, grocery shopping, and transporting Rani, who did not have a license to drive. Rani's son did the lawn work. Although some small group homes are owned and operated by companies, Valley Glen truly represents the family-style approach.

The Residents

At our first visit to Valley Glen Home in the spring of 2002, five women, ranging in age from 79 to 95, lived there. In addition to Rani's mother and Miss Helen, the other residents were Rosalie, Nellie, and Iveris. Rosalie showed little dementia but had severe arthritis that affected her ability to walk. Nellie, experiencing fairly advanced dementia, had been in four senior housing settings before her daughter and a private case manager placed her at Valley Glen. At that time she could talk, but she reverted to her native German before losing the ability to talk, walk, or feed herself. Similarly, Iveris, a six-year resident, now spoke only a few sporadic phrases, mostly in Spanish. All but one of these residents was incontinent. This level of limitation among the residents required a great deal of care and supervision on the part of Rani and her employees. The workers could not rely on any resident other than Rosalie to be able to ask for assistance with any necessary task. Instead, they had to anticipate and observe the daily needs of these elderly women.

During the 11 months of our fieldwork, one of the original residents died and two additional residents (both women) moved in: Jane, who had mild memory loss, and Lucille, who was recovering from a recent fall and hospitalization. Rani told us that before admitting new residents she attempted to make certain that they were not at risk of "wandering" out of the house and did not have behavioral problems such as aggression. However, Rani learned too late that these two new residents each fit one of these categories.

Jane seemed to have fairly mild memory loss when Rani evaluated her, and her family assured Rani that Jane would remain in the house. But in fact she did walk out on two occasions, resulting in several anxiety-filled hours for Rani and Jane's family until she was found. Assisted living managers often rely on relatives of prospective new residents to provide information on medical conditions, habits, preferences, and behaviors such as wandering. While some managers believe that families intentionally misrepresent their relative's abilities to get them admitted, Rani thought that most likely Jane's family simply didn't expect that she would wander away.

The two new residents could not have been more different. While Jane was reserved and quiet, Lucille was highly verbal and demanding. Most days Jane was happy to have afternoon tea time, occasionally asking heartbreaking questions like, "Am I going to be here for all of my life?" Although Lucille, who was then 90, did not have a diagnosis of a cognitive impairment, she presented challenging behavioral issues, the result of chronic mental illness, resentment at being placed in a care home by a case manager, or a combination of these and other unknown factors. Lucille screamed and cursed profusely, refusing to leave her room yet not wanting to be left alone. She pondered aloud what would happen to the rest of her life; she advised the two field ethnographers that we should enjoy life now before it was too late: "Whatever you want to do, do it now."

The addition of these two women upset the previous calm of Valley Glen Home and was a strain on Rani, who attempted to spend as much time as possible with each of them as they adapted to life in assisted living. Rani provided highly individualized attention during what she called the "settling in" stage. She explained that when a new resident arrived, she would not leave the facility for at least a month to provide continuity.

Like most assisted living residents, neither Jane nor Lucille had much control over the decision to leave her prior home, nor about where or when to go. As Rani explained, "in group homes, the kind of people who come are not the ones who can decide things for themselves." This leaves the large list of choices about whether to move, into what type of place, when to move, how much to pay, and so on, up to families, who might also enlist the advice of paid professionals, doctors and nurses, clergy, and friends.

In Jane's case, her six children agreed that their mother needed assistance. They had been increasingly involved in her care since the death of Jane's husband five years before she moved to Valley Glen Home at age 80. Her daughter, Tammy, told us that over time, as Jane's memory and cognitive abilities declined, they hired people to help Jane in her home for several hours a day. Jane did not like having "strangers" in her home, nor did she want to live with any of her relatives. She knew that her mind wasn't what it used to be and told her children, "I'm so confused, it's time for you to put me in a home."

Like Miss Helen's daughter, Alicia, Tammy finally hired a private firm that specialized in locating senior housing. She took this step after Rosemary, the person who came to evaluate Jane, said that Jane would soon need someone with her 24 hours a day and suggested assisted living residences. The six children divided up a list of places to visit, and Tammy explained that it was "good advice from Rosemary to start looking as early as we did. Because the first time you do it, it is such a shock. To think of Mom going from—she is living in a whole house—to going to that little tiny room—very much of a shock!" They looked at new large buildings with flower-filled foyers, at older buildings, and at small homes, and they easily agreed that smaller was better because they were concerned that their mother would get lost trying to find the dining room in a large building.

The first weeks after Jane's family brought her to Valley Glen Home were confusing for her, but her children, grandchildren, and brother organized a schedule so that at least one relative would be there to see her each day. Even though Jane quickly forgot that anyone had been to see her or had taken her out to eat, the family believed it was important that someone be there. Rani, too, was committed to helping Jane as Jane repeatedly pondered "Where am I?" and "Why am I here?" Rani explained that all new residents need to be told that they are in a safe place and that everything will be all right, but that Jane would likely need daily reassurance because of her memory loss. Although Jane was confused, she remained pleasant and accommodating.

Lucille, on the other hand, was not happy about moving to Valley Glen Home, and she focused her sizeable anger on Rani. Lucille came to Valley Glen from a hospital after she fell from her bed during the middle of the night and was not found until the next day. She had an emergency alert system but forgot to use it. Although she suffered only bruising, it was the last straw. She had lived in a high-rise apartment building for several years, and as her health declined during her eighties, her only known relative, a niece who lived in another state, arranged for and paid a private case manager to check in on Lucille. Sara, a trained social worker, was employed by a private geriatric case management firm. She regularly visited Lucille, and she hired a caregiver for a few hours a week to make certain that Lucille had food, saw a doctor, took her medications, and paid her bills.

Over time, Lucille's increasing frailty and memory loss resulted in several scares. The fall from her bed convinced Sara, if not Lucille, that it was time to move Lucille to assisted living. Sara told Lucille that the move would be temporary, just until she recovered, even though she secretly planned to cancel the lease on Lucille's apartment. About this ruse, Sara said: "When we move people we give them as much information as they can handle. And with her, we never talked about—your apartment is gone and all your stuff is gone and this is it. And so she would always refer back to—I mean it took her several months before she would stop asking about her apartment and paying the rent, and paying all the utilities and different bills and things like that. It took a while to let go of that."

Lucille's transition was traumatic for nearly everyone at Valley Glen. She shouted obscenities at Rani and the direct care workers; she repeatedly screamed, "God take me now; I want to die!" causing at least one other resident to join in with similar pleas. Rani said that Lucille's attitude spread to the others "like a poison." To further complicate matters, Lucille's health deteriorated, and she was hospitalized for a bowel obstruction. A home health nurse and nutritionist visited her when she returned to Valley Glen and strategized with Rani and Sara about how best to get Lucille to eat more, as she was losing weight. Sara, knowing about Lucille's sweet tooth, brought chocolate-flavored nutrition drinks and cookies. Despite Rani's best efforts to please Lucille, Sara reported to us that Lucille told Rani: "I'm really glad I'm here. It's *you* I don't like."

Still, Rani worked to get to know Lucille and to meet her on her own terms while slowly acclimatizing her to living at Valley Glen. Lucille insisted on eating her meals in her room while watching television, a lifelong habit. Rani accommodated this wish but also bargained to get Lucille to have one daily meal with the others. Rani introduced Lucille to Rosalie, hoping that a friend would ease her distress. Over several weeks, Lucille did adjust despite complaining of a sore leg and ongoing stomach pains. In January, five months after moving to Valley Glen, Lucille suddenly collapsed at the dinner table, and Rani called an ambulance. Lucille died the following day of a heart attack; the suddenness of her loss was shocking to Rani, to her staff, and to Sara, the case manager. Only one resident, Rosalie, was capable of comprehending Lucille's departure; if the others were aware of this development, they did not show it and Rani chose not to tell them.

Even as new residents adapt to life in assisted living and much time and energy are focused on making necessary adjustments, the topic of aging in place comes up. For example, the staff and family might question whether the facility is or ever will be the right fit and for how long the individual might be able to stay. Jane's two unescorted journeys out of Valley Glen posed such questions because Rani's house did not have alarms to prevent someone from wandering out. Rani had to decide whether or not she could retain a resident who made repeated efforts to leave; she tentatively agreed to do so but only after locking Jane's bedroom window so that at least one possible escape route was controlled. Jane's family had to decide whether their mother might be better off in a dementia care facility that had alarms on the exits. Jane's daughter Tammy explained her feelings about this:

> I love [having my mother] with Rani and I want her to stay there with Rani. But you know—I don't want her to be locked up, even at Rani's. And Rani doesn't want the window open. And I want the window open. And I'll tell Rani, "I will take the responsibility if you want, I will write that down—if she climbs out the window and falls and breaks her neck—it's my responsibility—I will take that—she needs the window open." Obviously I don't believe Mother would do

it or I wouldn't go along with it—but I've talked to all my brothers and sisters and they are all in agreement too —"That's right, if she falls out—so be it—you know we did the best we could." When she got out the last time, I said, "Rani, you are going to have to tell me when this is no longer the right place for her. Unless it's obvious to me, I would rather keep her here." So I said, "You are going to have to say when her care is just getting beyond you." And I told her then—"If you want, I'd pay for another aide just to keep her here."

Fortunately, Jane did adjust to life at Valley Glen and no longer attempted to leave on her own. Her children, too, adjusted to their mother's new life and capabilities. They learned that taking her out for drives or to a restaurant were too confusing for her; she did better with a small number of visitors and with phone conversations. Even so, they prepared themselves for eventual change by gathering information on dementia care facilities should they need to move Jane yet again.

The Employees

Rani described herself as "resident manager or assisted living assistant or something like that." Her explanation might be seen as a lack of pretense and a subtle disregard for the state's official terminology ("assisted living manager"). When we began our research at Valley Glen, she employed two staff members, both women, both from Africa (Tanzania and Zambia). Matilda attended college on the weekends and had worked at Valley Glen Home for several months, living there during the week. Grace lasted only two weeks and was replaced by Yolanda, who was from West Africa and had worked on and off for Rani since 1996.

Both Rani and her sister, Priya, reported that staffing, including finding individuals with the right attitude and abilities, presented an ongoing challenge. They preferred to hire live-ins but only rarely found an individual willing to accept such a lifestyle. More often, they hired three round-the-clock shifts, but it sometimes happened that Rani was by herself at night, the only one available to respond if any of the residents in her care awoke needing assistance. This situation was permissible by state rules and was supported by the use of baby monitors to better hear sounds in resident rooms. Maryland continues to debate a requirement for "awake overnight staff," a rule that would apply to all assisted living settings regardless of whether there are 5 or 105 residents but would have greater fiscal impact on small homes with limited staffing.

Rani and Priya had both completed certified nursing assistant (CNA) training, and after completing medication management coursework, Rani took sole responsibility for administering each resident's daily medications. She told us that she worried that an employee, especially a newer one, would make a mistake. Both women took continuing education courses from a county agency and from a senior housing trade group to bolster their skills and understanding of the changing context of assisted living. The training schedule of the senior housing trade group did not fit Rani's schedule very well because as one of usually only two staff members there at any given time, she was rarely able to leave Valley Glen Home during the day. In any case, Rani told us that the care she had provided to elderly relatives in India provided her with the best knowledge about how to assist her residents.

Over the years, some of her employees completed CNA training, some were nursing students, others had worked as home health aides, and a few had no prior caregiving experience. Matilda, the aide from Tanzania, had cared for her own family members and viewed it as a normal part of life. She said that when her grandmother came to live with her family, her own mother had prepared her for three-generational living by telling Matilda and her siblings, "You should remember. She is learning to live with you as much as you are learning to live with her." Matilda extended this sensitivity to the residents of Valley Glen Home, realizing that she was "the one that needs to change and suit this environment" to make their lives comfortable.

Regardless of each person's prior experience, Rani provided on-the-job training for new employees. She told us that it sometimes worked best if a new hire did not have prior medical training because then she could teach that person to do things the way she wanted them done rather than retraining him or her. She described her hands-on approach: "Initially I have to get myself involved a lot. In fact, every moment I am with new employees in the beginning. But if they are here for the next six months, say, then they get settled. They get to know the person [resident] and so they know how each one will react and what they require and so on. So when they get to know them then I am confident that they can take care of them, and then, at that point, I slowly try to withdraw. But initially, I have to make sure that everything goes on well and they know what to do with each person and with each situation."

Rani also spoke of the stress that some residents experience when employees quit, call in sick, or have transportation problems, leaving her short-staffed. In such cases, she might have to hire an aide from a private agency. Maintaining staffing consistency, she said, was the most difficult aspect of operating an assisted living home. She knew that ultimately she represented the main source of stability and continuity to the residents, especially to those with cognitive impairments, and for this reason, she rarely left the home.

Staffing decisions at Valley Glen Home were based on finances, training, and the needs of residents. Over time the residents' needs increased, and with this came added demands on Rani. For example, at one time she did not require staff assistance during the late afternoon hours because she was able to serve dinner to all of her residents, most of whom were able to get to the table and feed themselves. However, both Miss Helen and Nellie came to require help with eating and walking, so Rani had to hire staff on a 24-hour basis, at a significant additional cost.

In a small setting like this one, each employee contributes in many ways. The workers did not have formal titles; Matilda simply referred to herself as an "assistant." Rather than being specialized into work categories like direct care, housekeeping, and dining staff (among other categories found at some larger assisted living settings), the staff at small homes assist residents with personal care, do the laundry and housekeeping, prepare and serve meals, and provide emotional support, entertainment and activities, a hand to hold, and many other counted and uncounted tasks.

Valley Glen Home: Group Home or Assisted Living?

When Valley Glen Home opened for business in the fall of 1995, it was designated as a group home according to the classification system in effect in the state at that time. The regulations governing senior housing, in Maryland as in other states, seem always to be in transition (Mollica, Johnson-Lamarche, and O'Keeffe 2005; OHCQ 2005). Rani continued to use the term "group home" to describe Valley Glen, despite the state's implementation of the assisted living licensure category two years before our first meeting with her. The differences between traditional group homes—many with three or fewer residents (Morgan, Eckert, and Lyon 1995)—and contemporary assisted living homes range from the trivial to the profound. The regulatory climate in Maryland and other states means that small homes maintain a tenuous hold within the larger world of "assisted living" (Carder, Morgan, and Eckert 2008). What these small homes are called might matter less than whether or not they are seen as legitimate long-term care alternatives in the eyes of policymakers and consumers.

As a licensed assisted living setting, Valley Glen Home participated in the Medicaid subsidy program, received technical support from agency staff, qualified for liability insurance, and most importantly, received referrals from agency staff on behalf of potential clients. Miss Helen's daughter, Alicia, chose Valley Glen for her mother in part because of the strong recommendation from a county agency employee. However, these positive aspects of being licensed as an assisted living residence were counterbalanced by the strings of regulations.

Many operators dread the various inspections (e.g., state licensure agency, fire marshal) that periodically interrupt the regular flow of daily life and care. Given the relatively long list of regulatory items that each assisted living facility has to enact, record, and oversee, the potential that an inspection will uncover some problem looms large. Rani told us that, from her experience, the meanings of particular regulations seemed to change from one visit to the next. For example, the state regulations permit "capable residents" to administer their own medications if there is space to store and lock medications within their apartment or room. But at one visit to Valley Glen a state regulator took Rani by surprise by focusing on over-the-counter medications kept in the residents' rooms, as Rani told the ethnographer:

> Rani said she had prepared all the files and all the paperwork was in impeccable order, the place was clean, everything was ready. But this time they checked the creams and lotions in everybody's room. Rani was miffed and frustrated. Nellie has a lotion in her room, placed where she cannot get to it. [Nellie could not walk.] The lotion was there for the caregivers to apply to Nellie's skin each night. . . . And what about Rosalie? The inspector asked if she could look inside

Rosalie's dresser drawers, and Rosalie said, "No." Apparently the inspector opened the drawers anyway and found some creams that she applies to her legs when they hurt. This application of arthritis creams for her knees is something Rosalie can do for herself. Rani is incensed. "Now I am supposed to make Rosalie ask for it every time she wants it?!"

This example highlights the contradiction that sometimes occurs in assisted living facilities between supporting a resident's independence, creating a strategy that meets the needs of residents and care staff, and the definition of risk. Rani once explained that "the county tells us . . . we have to help the residents to maintain their independence and whatever they can do they should be able to do as much as they can. So we try to do that." Yet now she was penalized for allowing one cognitively capable resident to keep medicated lotions in her room and for leaving medicinal cream in the room of Nellie, who was incapable of independent movement. Rani argued that her residents were not at risk of ingesting the substance in question and that the regulation made life less convenient for all involved. She did not mention the possibility of providing a locked cabinet to store the medicines in residents' rooms, as the regulations would have permitted.

Rani's kindhearted desire to provide for the needs of her residents conflicted with the state requirements in other ways. For example, she described how she once determined what Rosalie needed: "She has a sensitive stomach. Digestion is a bad problem with her. So I used to discover what is good for her and what is not good and give her what was right. . . . So I used to give her antacids. So I am telling you . . . we are not supposed to give any medication without a doctor's receipt—over the counter or anything. . . . But now, nobody told me she has the acid problem or the problems of digestion. . . . I just thought it was important to take care of her problem rather than to bother with, you know, some kind of regulation. So I gave her this antacid and then she felt better."

Rani went on to explain that she knew that heartburn could mask a more serious condition such as a heart attack, and she took care to monitor Rosalie's status. Although she had been trained to administer medications, Rani was permitted only to follow the directions on prescribed medications. It appeared that Rani took a more quasifamilial role in trying to do what seemed best for the health of those in her care, rather than a professional/medical approach that would have conformed more to the regulatory view. The extensive amount of time that Rani spent with each resident seemed to foster intimate and intuitive knowledge that transcended the regulatory assumptions that require mass solutions to individualized situations. Her attitude that the women under her care were "like family" might explain why she felt justified in administering common over-the-counter medications without a "doctor's receipt." Perhaps ironically, state regulations would permit Rani to make such medication decisions for her own mother, who lived in one room, but not for Rosalie, who lived in another nearby.

Another requirement that the new state assisted living rules imposed was a designation of each resident's "level of care." As a licensed manager, Rani needed to observe and record the medical diagnoses, physical abilities, and cognitive impairments of each resident. A state-developed form provided a checklist of items and a scoring system from 0 to 3. Level 1 described people who needed little assistance and level 3 those who needed a great deal. During the course of an interview, Rani first described Miss Helen as level 2 and then as level 3, with the explanation that Miss Helen "gets the maximum help that we can give, but on the behavioral aspects she is excellent. She has always been excellent. So, she is under level 2. But the amount of care we give is not level 2. We give her total care—we call it. We give her care for every aspect of her day-to-day living."

Several minutes later, Rani clearly separated the physical from the behavioral—perhaps a function of her training in psychology. Pointing out that the state level-of-care system has four levels, from 0 to 3, she said: "So earlier when Miss Helen came she was on 1 or 0, but now she is on 3. But when it comes to behavioral items she is the same."

So, was Miss Helen level 2 or 3? The apparent confusion became understandable when Rani explained her understanding of the state's level-of-care system. Referring to another resident, she said: "Now actually she is level 1, but she is assessed at level 2. Now, that's interesting because if you go under certain programs, like Medicaid waiver, they don't give Medicaid waiver for level 1. So, everyone who goes under that will have to be a 2. So when I was trying to assess, I have a problem to give numbers, because I can't say that she needs a whole lot of care. Because I know that she doesn't need, but it has to be according to the regulation set up there."

In short, there were cross-pressures between evaluating level of care realistically in terms of physical and cognitive traits and the funding that might—or might not—be available to retain residents in Valley Glen Home. In addition, there is tension between subjective and objective level-of-care measures. Rani described the care that she gave to Miss Helen as "total" (in regard to physical tasks such as eating, bathing, and using the toilet) and "very easy" (in the sense that she caused no trouble or disruption). Based on an objective functional assessment of Miss Helen—that is, the way she is presented on paper—it is safe to say that she would not be retained in many assisted living facilities (Chapin and Dobbs-Kepper 2001).

Most important, perhaps, is that to Rani, Miss Helen was more than the official record and more than a statistic; she was family. In describing the care that Rani and her assistants provide to Miss Helen and others, the daughter of another resident said, "They are attached. That's the thing. The staff love them, you know." This personally focused and quasifamilial approach to assisted living explains why subjective feelings and objective assessments merge into apparent uncertainty over whether Miss Helen is a level 2 or a level 3. In this case, a relational model of care affects decisions related to determining the level of care.

Final Thoughts

As Alicia reflected on her mother's physical and cognitive decline, she remarked, "I think if I wheeled her in as she is today, I don't know if Rani would have taken her." She described the deep relationships now shared between herself, her mother, Rani, and Rani's assistants that had developed over time. Alicia especially appreciated that Rani lived in the home with her own mother, believing that this arrangement resulted in long-term stability that could not be matched by most other settings. When Rani was asked to compare her home with other assisted living residences, she said, "We are different. Mainly because we interact with the residents so much more closer. In time we come to feel they are a part of us. We are a big family. That's how we feel, as time goes on."

Despite the family-like relationships, Rani had to make difficult choices about which residents could stay and which ones she might have to discharge. For example, she had to ask one resident to move after this resident, like Miss Helen, became incapable of walking and required total assistance to move between bed and wheelchair. The difference was one of scale. Miss Helen was small and relatively easy for Rani and one other person to lift. The other resident simply weighed more than two women could manage to lift on a daily basis, and Rani had to ask the woman's family to relocate her. This practical reality might not differ from that faced by family caregivers who place their relative in a skilled nursing home when the individual's condition exceeds the family's capacity to assist.

Cultures of Care

The operator has a large role in shaping the culture of a specific place. Above all, in spite of the various classifications and regulations that defined assisted living, Valley Glen Home was "Rani's Place." It is difficult to imagine her version of assisted living care being developed nationally into a chain of assisted living residences because it was so dependent on her style. Rani's approach was highly personal and relational; all the rest—the regulations, official titles, and standardized tools for classifying residents into levels of care—she simply dealt with as needed. Sometimes this approach conflicts with other cultures of care.

Senior housing and long-term-care regulators use concepts such as functional status, admission and discharge criteria, and levels of care when they define and enforce rules governing assisted living. Therefore, in addition to the local culture established by Rani, Valley Glen Home operates within a larger culture that relies on objective standards to define levels of care and admission and discharge criteria. Rani variously described Miss Helen's level of care as 2, 3, "total," and "very easy." These standard constructs, although required by regulations, miss many dimensions of daily practice, especially those that might fall under a relational model of care.

The experience of this study at Valley Glen Home might prompt us as researchers, policymakers, and practitioners to reexamine the rationale and value of basing policy and practice decisions solely on the status of individuals as represented by a numeric score. The case of Miss Helen at

Valley Glen asks us to question our assumptions. Clearly, statistics provide only part of the larger picture.

What is missed in the numeric level-of-care scores is the obvious fact that Miss Helen was loved by Rani, Matilda, and Yolanda. While assisted living regulations define a service called "grooming," the earlier description of the intricate and elegant braiding of Miss Helen's hair by an African caregiver, a process that would have taken well over an hour, clearly indicates that much more may be taking place.

THREE

Opal at Franciscan House

Maria [the owner-operator] takes us on a quick tour of Franciscan House. The front door opens onto the living room, where all but one of the residents is seated; everyone knows the comings and goings of anyone entering or leaving the house. Maria shows us the dining room, the kitchen, and a small powder room in the entrance hall. Off the entrance hallway there is a second downstairs hallway that leads to one resident room and to the room of the live-in caregiver, Angelina. Maria escorts us into the resident room without knocking. On a bed is a woman who seems to be just sitting, doing nothing. She is a bit gruff and says hello to us when we are introduced, although with no inflection in her voice and a bit of a scowl on her face. She is Opal. Maria leaves the room without shutting the door, and Opal comes to the door and demonstrably closes the door behind us. She seems to want to be left alone, not bothered.

Franciscan House, like Valley Glen Home, is one of the legions of anonymous small group homes scattered throughout the country. Located in a suburban community, this two-story house does not stand out from any other dwelling in the neighborhood. Yet it is a licensed business, a workplace, and a home to those who reside there, whether staff or paying customer.

Over the course of nine months of fieldwork in Franciscan House and three years of follow-up telephone calls, we witnessed both the stability of day-to-day life and the changes, including the addition of new residents and the death of others. Most of the seven older persons we found residing there on our first day of research had been there for at least two years, including Opal, who had arrived in 2000 and was still there at a follow-up in January 2007. During the time we knew her, Opal's ability to recall events, both distant and recent, became increasingly limited, and although she was able to make social small talk, she often argued with others at Franciscan House.

From Opal's experiences we learn some of the possibilities and limitations of a small group home. Opal was accepted despite her frequent verbal outbursts; she could shower herself with direction from Angelina but had no idea what kind of medication she took or for what conditions; and she was bored with watching television and wished for more meaningful activities. Her day-to-day routine represents the relative stability and ordinariness of everyday life in a small-group assisted living home.

Introducing Opal

Our understanding of Opal's story developed over nearly four years and is based on eight interviews with her, as well as interviews with Maria, Angelina, and the relatives of other residents. We identified Opal as a focal case in part because she is typical of the current cohort of assisted living residents; she was a widowed woman who worked at low-wage jobs while raising her children, and she showed signs of early dementia. Yet Opal was unique in other ways. At 75, she was younger than the other Franciscan House residents, whose ages ranged up to 87 (the average age was 83), and younger than the national average (NCAL 2007). She had worked as a licensed practical nurse until relatively late in her life and still referred to herself as a nurse. Finally, unlike the other residents described in this book, Opal was not particularly well liked by the staff, other residents, and their families. This relative "outsider" status led us to focus on her. We wondered how and why Franciscan House's owner, Maria, put up with her and how she affected daily life in this small home. Although Opal might not be the typical assisted living resident in all dimensions, there doubtless are other individuals like her who live in these residences somewhat uneasily, at times creating conflict and at other times fitting in as part of the group.

Opal tended to converse in small talk, commenting on the weather or what she or others were wearing. At times she related convincing details about her childhood, college, her marriage to a military man, and her children. And yet, in response to a question about the happiest event in her life, she stated, "I'm sure there was a lot of them, but I can't remember." (This comment came at the end of a 90-minute interview during which she described many happy events, including a "wonderful" marriage and four children.) Was this response due to fatigue after a long interview, uncertainty about how to answer an overly broad question, or a sign of dementia? Earlier in the interview she said: "I don't remember much of anything. See that's my biggest problem is my memory is going really fast. I don't remember when I did things." While she could not recall how long she had lived at Franciscan House, she could describe the other residents (though not by name) and the daily routines. Opal didn't know the name "Franciscan House" but knew that she did not care for Maria, whom she sometimes referred to as "that lady out there."

Most of what Opal said seemed plausible, but not everything did. For example, she said that her children took her car from her because they thought she was too old to drive. But then she added that they put the car into a river. Not unlike other people we interviewed, she retold several stories during our conversations, including the death of her husband, her mother, and her brother. But in one telling of her mother's death, Opal remained in Germany, where her husband was stationed, because she didn't think that she should leave her children. In a later telling of this story, she implied that she cared for her mother throughout her illness. Maria once noted about Opal that, "You wouldn't know that she has dementia." Over time, however, Opal's memory loss became increasingly evident to her and to others, though she remained in good physical health during the time that we followed her life at Franciscan House.

We identified two themes that seem to influence the way Opal lived her life inside this assisted living setting. Much of what we know about Opal's life revolved around conflict with others, including employers and family, and then with Maria and the other residents. The second theme, "It's the most boring life you can imagine," describes her attitude toward living at Franciscan House.

A Lifetime of Conflict

Opal often described conflicts that occurred throughout her life. Although she had a happy childhood, her family was "lucky sometimes just to have flour for biscuits." She grew up in Mississippi during the Depression, graduated from high school when she was 17, and then completed nursing school. Her husband was a local boy who joined the military; after their marriage, they moved several times, eventually living on two southern military bases and in Germany.

Opal said that she had a "real good marriage," but that her husband died after 12 years, leaving her to care for their four children. She regretted an unresolved argument with her husband shortly before his death. She explained that they did not typically fight but that she had been angry with him on that day. Opal married a second time, but this marriage lasted less than one year because "it was terrible conditions." So she raised four children by working as a licensed practical nurse and with financial support from her husband's military pension. Opal's discussion of her more recent history was murky compared with the rich detail she offered about her younger years. She explained that over time she lived with her son, brother, and/or one of her three daughters. It is likely that she did spend some time living with each of these family members.

What remained consistent was some form of conflict with each person; these conflicts resulted in her living alone later in life, something she did not like. In particular, she hated eating alone. Possibly the most dramatic conflict she described was an exchange with one of her daughters sometime before moving to Franciscan House: "We almost come into a fight; I twisted her arm, and she twisted my arm, like this you know, and I got mad because it was a bad twist, and I left. I should have stayed there." Even after this event, Opal continued to wonder whether it might still be possible for her to live with this daughter rather than at Franciscan House. Although we do not have data to suggest whether physical battles like the one described here were common in Opal's life, during an assessment interview, she volunteered, "Sometimes I'd like to hit people; I'd like to hit the woman that owns this place." To our knowledge, she never carried through with this thought.

Opal's history of conflict followed her into Franciscan House, where she regularly had heated verbal exchanges with Maria and with the other residents. The daughter of one resident described Opal as "nasty." Maria explained, "So far I'm blessed, except for Opal. She just has her own temper." Opal herself said, "I usually get along pretty good with people. Of course, I don't get along with these people here very much. I don't dislike them, but I don't like them either and I think there's a difference in that." Another time she summed up her personality by saying, "I'm not the friendliest person; not friendly, but I'm not unfriendly either." Opal's unwillingness to interact with others meant she lived essentially alone in a home the size of a typical suburban house with seven other residents and a live-in caregiver.

Opal described herself as someone who always did what she wanted to do; from her perspective, living in a small residential setting like Franciscan House clearly conflicted with her former life. She said: "Maria's boss here, and you gonna know she's boss. And so, the other things that she does and goes through, or she ever has to say anything about it, you won't do it again. So, it works pretty well, because if you had, I had an argument with one of the girls [referring to another resident], Nancy here, very big, but Maria didn't get involved in it, she just let it, me and Nancy argue until we'd argued out. So, I've got no argument about this place or with Maria." (Nancy had a close relationship with Tom, the only male resident of Franciscan House; the two typically sat next to each other on the living room couch, often holding hands. Opal often spoke of wanting Tom's attention, and this was an ongoing source of friction between the two women.)

Opal's outspoken manner challenged Maria's commitment to stability and routine at Franciscan House. Maria attempted to implement an efficient schedule and a home managed through routines that included getting each resident up and dressed before serving breakfast, as she explained in an interview: "Like some of the residents, they said, 'We want to eat first before we get dressed,' so we give into that. But then eventually we say, 'See, all the girls are dressed up so nicely, why don't you try to,' [and] eventually they do that too. It's contagious when they see that they are so odd compared to the rest. They would, like Opal used to say, 'No, I eat first before I take a shower,' but then afterwards, I say, 'Okay, breakfast is not ready yet so take a shower, everybody is done, you're next, you're the last one.' So she would just give in and do that. Eventually they blend in. But to start with they have their own personality."

Opal confirmed Maria's need for stability: "It's always been the same," she said. "That woman that runs the place here, you know, she always makes it the same." These comments illustrate the boundaries of individuality and autonomy in a small group setting, almost like a large family that requires some semblance of order to avoid sliding into chaos. Although Opal apparently adjusted to Maria's schedule, through challenging the routines she often got her own way. For example, Maria preferred that the residents remain in the living room during the day; all of them did so except for Opal, who most often stayed in her room either reading or simply sitting on her bed. Maria may have accepted this compromise because of her discomfort with Opal's occasional outbursts. Conflicts arose from tangible events, such as an episode when another resident sat in Opal's preferred living room chair, as well as disagreements that were less obvious to others. When Opal did join the others, her presence was heard and felt as she made demands for a specific food or drink or for something to do, or told the others what they should be doing. Maria often permitted Opal to keep to herself as a way of maintaining the peace.

"It's the Most Boring Life You Can Imagine"

Even though Opal once described Franciscan House as a nice place to live, she most often spoke of the unending boredom, and she repeated this theme during each of her interviews. Some of the tedium resulted from her perception that there was nothing worthwhile to do. Opal had always worked: "By 10 years old I was out there getting the milk and getting vegetables and going and selling, selling to the people around the neighborhood." She said she would have liked to cook a meal on occasion, but Maria would not permit it.

Opal's main form of enjoyment came from reading. She liked to read the newspaper because then, "you're not just dumb about what goes on in the world." She expressed a desire to keep up with current events, both locally and abroad, and she wished that the others at Franciscan House could have discussions based on magazines and news events. The other residents were too cognitively impaired to do so—and possibly Opal was as well. She also said that she would go to church if given the chance, and she thought Maria should take the residents. But in fact Maria arranged for a local minister to visit each month to give a sermon. Opal chose not to listen to him because "he's not the kind of preacher I like, anyway."

Opal spoke of many other things she would do if given the chance: go camping, go dancing or to a movie, take a college class, join a book group, go bowling, go to a senior center, go shopping, go to the library, and get married to "a nice man." Her life choices were constrained in part because Franciscan House offered only a few activities (e.g., bingo, music), most of which Opal refused to join, and because of her meager finances. She relied on public subsidies to pay her monthly fee; the small stipend did not permit her to purchase anything more than basic personal items, such as toiletries. Few of the larger assisted living settings in Maryland, the ones most likely to offer a full menu of social activities, accepted individuals who relied on public subsidies.[1]

During the time we knew her, Opal first shared a room with Lucy. After Lucy died she shared with Mildred, who was deaf and nearly blind. Maria provided the furnishings in this and all rooms throughout the house. Opal's room contained two twin beds, each with a dark wooden headboard, and a side table on which sat a brass lamp. The matching bedspreads displayed a wild print with large pink tropical flowers and pink ruffles. The two beds were positioned parallel to each other, with either headboard flanking a window, through which a large shade tree was visible. At the foot of each bed was an upholstered chair, and on the wall over each bed was a wooden cross adorned with dried fronds from a Palm Sunday church service. Each resident had at least one framed picture of family members located on the wall or a side table, a wooden bureau of drawers, and a closet. The floor was covered in a low-nap dark brown carpet, and the walls were painted a warm cream color. Unlike some other assisted living settings, the furnishings of rooms included few items from former homes reflective of the personality or history of the individuals sleeping there.

Opal was not the only person to observe that life at Franciscan House was often dull. Most of the residents' families felt generally positive about the care received by their relatives, but some with whom we spoke complained about the lack of activities. The residents spent most of their time sitting around watching television. Maria sometimes led the residents in song or word games as well as seated stretching exercises, but the small living room left little space for other pastimes. In addition, most of Maria's time was devoted to keeping the home organized and operating smoothly, with tasks including cleaning, purchasing groceries, completing state-mandated paperwork, and making certain that each resident remained healthy and physically stable.

Franciscan House was opened in 1989 by Maria and Phillip Agbuya, a couple originally from the Philippines. At first they lived at Franciscan House with their two children, but they later moved the family into a nearby single-family home. Their approach to running a group home differed from that used by Rani at Valley Glen Home. The Agbuyas clearly separated their family life from the business of providing care to the residents, in contrast to Rani, who lived in the home with her own mother and son. Maria's prior experience as an engineer probably guided her daily efforts to instill order, efficiency, and stability at the same time that her strong Catholic faith influenced her approach to caring for others, as we describe in more detail below.

Maria maintained responsibility for day-to-day operations, while Phillip, a registered nurse employed at a local hospital, assessed the residents' health care needs in addition to maintaining the lawn and a terraced garden behind the house. Angelina, the live-in caregiver (also from the Philippines), was responsible for personal care, housekeeping, laundry, and meal preparation. The Agbuyas moved to the United States with the hope that their teenaged children would get a better education and to be closer to Phillip's sister, who suggested that operating a group home would provide a good source of income. Paid caregiving for strangers was a foreign concept to Maria, as was the existence of "senior housing." In her home country, families cared for their frail relatives.

The research notes from the first visit to Franciscan House describe the neighborhood:

> Franciscan House is located in what seemed to be an unlikely suburban neighborhood of midsized two- to three-bedroom homes, mostly bi-level. The neighborhood was thoroughly residential, without any neighborhood access to public transportation, shops, services of any kind. I would guess that homes in the neighborhood were built in the 1970s—a subdivision in the middle of nowhere carved out of field and pasture. The house had light tan aluminum siding, a car in the driveway, a garbage can and recycle bin neatly parked beside the driveway, a tidy lawn, an all-season wreath on the door, and no sign whatsoever that the residence was in any way different from all the other residences on the street. There

was no wheelchair access ramp at the front door (and none at the back), no sign identifying the place as an assisted living facility.

Franciscan House was located in a suburb of Washington, DC, that had a distinctly small-town flavor, with only 20,000 residents and a main street with shops and restaurants. The house had two bathrooms, one on the first floor, and the second upstairs, shared by the four female residents. All but two residents shared a bedroom. Maria once told us that she would have purchased a single-story house if she had known in advance the problems a two-level structure would present. For example, she could neither admit nor retain individuals who could not negotiate the stairs, even though she did install a stair lift. This was one reason that Maria worked diligently to preserve each resident's health and functional capacity—she wanted to retain them as residents for as long as possible.

Like Valley Glen Home, Franciscan House was licensed for eight residents and accepted public-subsidy clients. Four of the residents during our research there received this subsidy, administered by a county agency, to cover the basic costs of their care. Maria charged an additional monthly fee to cover room and board; some subsidy residents used Supplemental Security Income (SSI) payments to pay this cost, and others received support from their families. Most of the residents had mild to moderate dementia, but with one exception they were physically mobile and could dress themselves with prompting from Maria or Angelina.

In addition to Opal, there were six other residents at the time of our first meeting. Mildred was deaf and nearly blind, and had significant dementia. She did not have family; a legal representative paid her monthly bills but did not visit her. Nancy had a diagnosis of Alzheimer's disease but had been stable for three years; her two daughters lived nearby and were very much involved with their mother's life at Franciscan House. Christina had arrived with a diagnosis of possible malnutrition; Maria proudly reported that, within a few months, Christina had gained 30 pounds. Lucy moved from independent senior housing after she fell and injured herself; her granddaughter visited her each week. Tom had lived alone after his wife died, with his son checking on him. Over time he became increasingly confused and did not eat regular meals, so his family decided that he needed the kind of daily supervision provided in assisted living. Fern's son arranged to move his mother to Franciscan House because she, like Tom, lived alone and was increasingly confused, possibly due to poor nutrition. Although Fern had several children and had raised her sister's children, she received no visitors and rarely left the assisted living setting. Maria complained that the family did not respond to her requests to take Fern to the doctor and to get her medications, but the son who had moved Fern into Franciscan House was himself in poor health.

On most days, a sense of monotonous calm and tranquility reigned at Franciscan House. Phillip said that the "peace" derived from familiarity between Maria and the residents. During our visits, we witnessed days when the residents were social, talking with each other and Maria or Angelina, and other days when everyone seemed quiet. The conversations were never very deep, perhaps a product of dementia symptoms for many, although people did talk of their home, family, and work memories. Overall, these seven residents seemed disconnected, as though they were not fully aware that they lived in this home. On some of our visits, the living room environment felt more like a group of people sitting in a doctor's office waiting room. In fact, Tom sometimes mentioned that he was waiting for someone to pick him up.

Maria or Angelina occasionally led games of bingo, residents often watched the Lawrence Welk show or other musical programming, and Angelina liked to involve everyone in singing hymns reflective of her Catholic faith ("Jesus Loves Me" was popular with several residents). A mobile library unit visited every six weeks or so, and a podiatrist visited every nine weeks to trim nails and examine feet. Other than these minor events, each day was much like the one before. The residents had their usual places to sit in the living and dining rooms, probably partly by their own choice and partly because that was Maria's way of keeping things orderly.

Three themes seemed to define Franciscan House: the importance of order, running a business, and the moral code "Do unto others."

The Importance of Order

Aside from the six elderly residents seated in the living room in front of the TV and the stair lift on the stairs leading to the second floor, this could have been any other American home. It was clean—so clean that the floor squeaked under-foot. All was orderly, tidy, in place, and "ready."

Maria expected the residents to adapt to her schedule, though she made some minor accommodations. When asked if she would allow a resident to sleep in until 10 a.m., she said, "No, we get them. Sometimes we do say, 'It's almost quarter to nine. You better get up now,' you know. We just change the time a little. But when they hear the time, then they will get up. Or we say, 'Coffee is hot. You're going to get down late. Coffee is going to get cold.' I always tell them, 'Coffee is ready, it's hot.' They like the smell of coffee."

Routine was important to Maria, who believed it benefited the residents, especially those with cognitive impairment. When one new resident moved in and went about his own way of doing things, including staying up late and then calling a cab and leaving without informing her, Maria was overwhelmed and asked him to move out after only a few days. Another time she explained, "A bad day is when there is just . . . when there is an accident like bowel movements—then the schedule is thrown off."

Maria's sense of order and routine applied not only to the daily schedule, but also to the care and medical oversight provided to Opal and the other residents. While she took responsibility for overseeing day-to-day care, Phillip formally evaluated each resident's medical condition at least every six weeks. Beyond these state-required evaluations, however, Phillip checked in on the residents each week. On these visits, he was available to discuss and answer Maria's questions about each resident's condition.

Keeping the peace in such a small space—basically a single-family home with eight adults residing in it—was critical to maintaining order and routine. Opal clearly challenged Maria's sense of order and routine, yet Maria did not ask her to move out. Keeping Opal as a resident was not related to money, because Maria could have charged a private-pay client much more.

Running a Business

From Maria we learned that the business of assisted living was hard work, that it required an intimate knowledge of each resident's condition, and that understanding and following the state and county rules and regulations created an added challenge for a small, solo operator. When asked to describe "one thing" that people should understand about Franciscan House and small group homes in general, Maria said, "Well, like in my experience, like I have seen people come here, they think this is an easy job. Okay, because everything seems to be so neat. All of the residents are clean, okay. They just pass by and they say, 'Oh, it's easy.' But I think it is not as easy as they think. Because you would have to stay here and live with them and then you would know what this really entails. If you love this type of job, I think it is really nice. . . . I enjoy it, but there are bad days, too. I can say like I'm not a perfect person. There are good and bad days, but generally I'm okay. . . . It has been 13 years almost. Aside from that, I think like people have to experience it. It's really a different type of work."

Maria chose to operate a group home (and then an assisted living residence as Maryland regulations changed) as a business decision and found it to be a good, though challenging, way to earn money. To prepare for opening Franciscan House, Maria and Phillip visited one assisted living residence, applied to the state regulatory agency for a license, and in two months became certified as providers. It was two more months before their first two residents moved in; both of them had been diagnosed with Alzheimer's disease. It was not easy, as Maria explained: "So I did the job. At nighttime I was so thankful Safeway was open for 24 hours. I went to the grocery store at night. It was hard. It was hard. Everything was hard, I mean. No pain, no gain. But we survived and then the kids, they went to school." Here she referred to the ultimate reason for her sacrifice: earning an income that would permit her two children to attend good colleges.

Maria was acutely aware of each resident's physical and mental status, and she worked to keep the residents in stable health by observing their eating habits, weight, blood pressure, and other vital signs. She explained: "If they are healthy, it makes my job easy." This focus on stability resulted in long-term residents at Franciscan House. Maria once noted that the census of residents tended to turn over every three years, and we observed this to be the case. About the residents, she said: "As long as they eat good, I never worry. The daily routine, it's just very stable. I don't know, I don't see such a big fluctuation. I don't know why, but it seems that they are very stable. Maybe I'm just blessed with the right residents. It's just that the residents that I have, even if they are up in age . . . 89, they seem to be very stable."

Franciscan House was licensed by the state of Maryland as a level 2 assisted living facility. To Maria, being licensed as level 2 meant that she admitted and retained only those residents with the ability to walk to the bathroom and stand in the shower: "When they cannot really walk to the bathroom, or I cannot shower them, when they become so stiff that I cannot handle it, I tell the family, it's time"—time, that is, for the resident to move out. However, she worked hard to maintain each resident to forestall decline that would lead to a move out of the facility.

Maria's preferred approach to her work was logical, rational, and orderly. Visits from regulators, such as the licensing agency, were often highly upsetting to her, in part because the different public employees who came to her home took different approaches to interpreting the requirements, and Maria could not cope with this lack of predictability. She often complained about the increase in paperwork following the adoption of assisted living regulations. After failing to pass an annual recertification inspection in the fall of 2002 because she did not keep "care notes" the way a regulatory department employee wanted, she said: "I think since the year 2000, everything has changed. All the rules, everything has changed and we are under the umbrella of the nursing homes. Whatever pertains to them, we have to comply, and I think it is hard on us. Before the year 2000, the rules were not as strict, okay, like they didn't ask for too many things. Now we have so many paperworks. We have to send this to the doctor. We have to do our own assessment. We didn't have that before. We have to have a 45-day nursing assessment and then we have so many reports like everything has to be documented just for the record, maybe because of so many lawsuits, I don't know. Every little thing we have to like write it down and send it to this form and send that form over there. It's too much."

The financial side of operating this small business was also an ongoing concern. Maria charged a monthly fee of $1,600 to the three private-pay residents, a rate much lower than the national average of $2,905 for basic services (MetLife 2005). Nancy's daughter told us: "I mean, they care about her. It isn't about money at Franciscan House. I mean, how they even do it is a mystery to me. It's like, God, you need to charge more!" When Fern's son stopped paying the full monthly charge, Maria told us that she would not put Fern "on the street," but she continued asking Fern's son to pay the full monthly fee. A dramatic rise in the cost of liability insurance during our research at Franciscan House and the other assisted living residences placed another financial burden on Maria, as she explained several times during our meetings with her.

As with most other businesses, success in operating an assisted living facility depends on hiring and training staff. Maria preferred to have a live-in caregiver, and she was successful in finding and retaining long-term employees. Angelina started work two months before our fieldwork began and remained throughout; the woman who was her predecessor at Franciscan House stayed for nearly six years.

Angelina was committed to her church and her faith. She had moved to the United States in 1996 with an American family for whom she had provided child care. She learned about Franciscan House through a church friend. Angelina explained that her daily routine included rising early to pray, then assisting two residents with a shower (a different two each day), helping people to use the toilet, getting breakfast prepared and served, turning on the television, making beds, doing laundry, and cleaning. She assisted Maria in preparing lunch and dinner, housekeeping, and all personal care. Maria was fully responsible for completing all of the paperwork, administering medications, and coordinating medical services with residents' families and physicians.

Maryland state regulations have only recently begun to require specific training for those who operate assisted living facilities. Employees come from many fields; some are certified nurse assistants (CNAs), while others receive on-the-job training. Assisted living managers like Maria and Rani tend to develop their own approaches to training the people they hire to do the bulk of the physical work. Maria did not try to teach Angelina everything at once, instead introducing specific tasks over several weeks' time. But Maria did impress on her employees the significance of their work. Maria once told us: "This is a big responsibility. I always tell my help, I say, 'I'm the one who is going to cut off my head if anything happens to them, so please if you don't know, you tell me. You have to be honest and tell me anything.' I mean it's not impossible for them to fall. They are right in front of you and they can trip with their toe and that's it, you know. So it's not impossible." Yet Maria worked hard to prevent accidents, in part by maintaining a routine and stable environment.

Maria's Catholic faith informed her approach to life and included a strong moral commitment to caring for others. When asked what it takes to be good at her job, she said, "I think it's just like some people say, it's a calling. That's the word they use. Or it's meant to be. I never knew I would be in this position. Like when I came to the United States, like I told you I'm a scientist. I just came in with no knowledge of patients, nothing. So, I guess it's just like more of instinct or an intuition. . . . The principle that guides me is . . . what I want others to do unto me, I do unto them, basically. So, I hope somebody will take care of me when I get old."

Although Maria did not refer to her residents as "family," she knew each one well and was especially attuned to maintaining their physical health. She and Angelina provided the bulk of daily care, but Maria also expected the residents' families to assist with transportation to medical appointments and related needs. She expressed frustration when a couple of family members did not respond to their relative's medical care needs. When Fern's family did not respond to her request to take her to the doctor, Maria became exasperated because she had informed the family in advance that she could not provide this service. Fern's acute skin condition needed immediate treatment, yet her family did not assist, leaving Maria to buy an over-the-counter ointment.

During one interview with us, Maria was asked to describe her top five concerns, and she listed family responsiveness as her second issue, after the high cost of prescription medications. Specifically, she said, "I think residents' families should spend more time when their parents are getting older because they have only a few years to live. But I don't see it [happen] that way. I see it that, as long as somebody is taking care of the parents, that's it. It's a sad thing." Certainly some of the family members were very involved, visiting on a weekly basis and taking the parent not only to medical appointments but also for social outings. One of Opal's daughters regularly took her out to eat and to get her hair styled. On the other hand, Mildred lacked family and left Franciscan House only to visit her doctor once or twice annually, and Fern's family did not take her out. Maria called the families to give them weekly, and sometimes daily, updates, and she expected them to be active in their parents' lives.

Most of the family members we spoke to in connection with Franciscan House residents were pleased with the care their relatives received. The daughter of one explained that she began by looking at large facilities but decided a small home would work best for her mother, who had dementia: "I was looking for somebody who would care for my mother, who would help bathe my mother, who would call me and tell me, my mother has a stomach ache or my mother has a headache or my mother has this ache. Those big homes aren't going to do that. You're not going to get a phone call, unless they are dead or injured. And that's what propelled us." So, although Franciscan House did not provide the social activities advertised in some of the larger assisted living settings, the small size and the continuity of care provided by Maria were appreciated. Research suggests that smaller settings benefit persons with cognitive impairments (Calkins 2001; Day, Carreon, and Stump 2000).

Final Thoughts

Franciscan House is largely hidden from society, with the daily work of caring for older persons quietly taking place within the walls of an average-looking home within a quiet suburban neighborhood. The main lessons to be learned from this particular setting and its culture are that maintaining stability requires rules and routines (both internal and external), that small homes sometimes provide "bored and care" (Dobkin 1989), and that small homes like this one seem to work especially well for individuals with mild cognitive impairment and good physical mobility.

From both Maria and Opal we learn that assisted living requires ongoing negotiations in which rules matter but can be bent and that lifetime patterns affect the quality of life. Maria operated a business licensed by a state agency and monitored by county agencies, and she had to comply with a large (and growing) set of regulatory requirements. Yet she also followed her own moral code to "do unto others," and this might have influenced her decision to retain Opal despite the low economic reward and relatively high emotional burden. Maria imposed her own standards to run the home in a way that she thought appropriate to maintain the health and physical function of each resident.

At our last interview with Opal in the spring of 2005, she remarked that we would not learn anything from her "because I'm kind of dull."

From Opal we hear that life inside a small assisted living setting can be "the most boring life you can imagine," but that this negative is balanced by benefits such as an affordable place to stay, people to talk to, and assistance when you need it. Despite the tedium of daily routines Opal said she was glad that she moved to Franciscan House.

While other small homes might provide more activities than this one, their type and quality will be constrained by the varying capacities (physical and mental) of residents and by the provider's concerns for liability. For example, Maria remarked that, in prior years when the current cohort of residents were more physically and cognitively capable, she would take them to church services, shopping, and out for lunch. Over time, Maria increasingly worried that one of them would fall and she would be sued, so she no longer took residents out, instead relying on families or public transit to provide this service. Over the many days and weeks of providing personal care to older persons, Maria and her husband came to know the kind of person they could best care for, and they worked hard to select individuals who would best fit the type of care they provided and then to provide a stable and secure living environment.

Update

After nearly 15 years operating a group home, Maria felt that the time was right for a change. Her aging parents, who lived in another state, were beginning to need assistance, and Maria's moral duty to "do unto others" included attending to her own parents. Her siblings had taken the primary responsibility thus far, and it was her turn. By now her two children were grown. The Agbuyas were proud of their engineer daughter and physician son; they had worked hard to provide the financial support to send them to college. Finally, the Agbuyas decided to sell Franciscan House. Their retirement plans include becoming certified hospice volunteers and traveling to other countries to do missionary work for their church.

FOUR

❀ Karen at Huntington Inn

Karen was the founder of "The Forum" at Huntington Inn, an unassuming cluster of five white plastic chairs that she talked a staff
member into placing in a wide section of the building's long hallway. Over
time, it became the regular meeting place for four or five residents as well
as a couple of staff members. During our research, we learned that it was
the place to go to catch up on the latest facility gossip. In addition to
Karen, the regular members of The Forum included Rose, who eventually
declined (or "gave up," as Karen said) to the point that she had to move
to a nursing home; Edith, the oldest resident at age 103; Donnie, a woman
who was disliked by nearly everyone but Karen; Lilleth, who had significant memory loss and often wore odd layers of clothes and mismatched
shoes; and Sylvia, who also had a poor memory, but could take part in
the social commentary, bantering, and discussion of health problems that
took place daily at The Forum.

Another resident, referred to as "Mother" by both the staff and the
residents, walked by The Forum several times a day as she paced to and
from the main entry with her baby doll (the reason for her nickname), and
tried to leave through the unlocked front door. Most of the residents, and
all of the staff, loved Mother; they would get her to smile by exclaiming
over the cuteness of her "baby." However, Mother eventually became the
source of a great deal of conflict among staff, residents, and family
members.

Karen told us she liked assisted living—"It's great!"—even though
she sometimes took issue with the policies, the administration, and the
food. A resident of 10 months at the time we met her in 2003, she described
Huntington Inn as her "home" and, when faced with being moved to a

nursing home because she had spent all of her savings, said, "I would hate to leave here."

In this chapter, we introduce Karen and Huntington Inn, and then provide details about daily life at this moderate-sized, rural assisted living residence. Through Karen's story, we learn how three major categories of change—finances, health, and public policies—affect the lives of those who live and work in this type of setting.

Introducing Karen

Karen, like many women in her generation (she was born in 1928), graduated from high school, married, then stayed home to raise her son. She took part-time low-wage jobs, such as school bus driver, dress salesperson, and cashier, while her only child, Mark, attended school.

Her favorite part-time job was as a veterinary assistant; Karen loved animals and said that she couldn't believe how lucky she had been to get paid for working with and cleaning up after them. When we interviewed Mark, he brought out a newspaper clipping from 1949 that included Karen's picture, mouth open wide, with a caption that read, "SPCA sympathizer." Karen sometimes talked about her desire to have a cat in her room at Huntington Inn, though she knew that it would be difficult to care for one. Besides, it was against the rules. However, the administrator had arranged for a volunteer pet program in which a woman visited about once a month with her two dogs. Some of the employees occasionally brought their own pets to visit on their days off work. Karen and other residents truly appreciated and looked forward to these visits.

After 52 years of what she described as an "abusive" marriage, Karen left her husband. (Mark said that the marriage was never physically abusive, only verbally so, and that the abuse went in both directions. He remained close to both his mother and father.) After the divorce, Karen lived for a short time with Mark but didn't want to intrude on his "bachelor lifestyle." Mark had never married, though he had a long-time girlfriend in a nearby city with whom he spent many weekends. During the short time that Karen lived at Mark's home, she fell and broke her hip. Though she did well in rehabilitation, Karen and Mark agreed that she needed to live in a place that gave her the social interaction and daily physical assistance she needed and where she could have her own space.

They considered Karen's situation: she didn't need ongoing nursing care and could independently manage the oxygen supplies she needed for emphysema. She could heat prepared food in a microwave or make a sandwich, but she could no longer drive. Her limited lung capacity made it difficult for her to take a shower or walk more than a few feet without assistance. It took her a long time to get dressed because she frequently had to stop to rest. Before moving to assisted living, she managed her own medications.

With the help of a friend of Mark's, they found Huntington Inn, located less than five miles away from Mark's apartment. Karen did not see her new home before moving in because she was in a rehabilitation center recovering from hip surgery. About her move she said, "When I came here from the hospital, I came at nine o'clock at night. Hadn't seen this place or knew about it or anything else. They brought me in an ambulance, took me out of the ambulance on a gurney. Mr. Hill was at the door waiting for us and he said, 'Put her in 18' and they rolled the gurney up the hall and put me in 18 and that was it."

Mr. Hill, the owner and "administrator" (his term) of Huntington Inn, took a hands-on approach to operating the facility. Most days he wore blue denim pants and a polo shirt because he never knew if he would be assisting a resident in the shower, tinkering with the laundry machine, or dealing with a plugged toilet—in addition to the paperwork, contacts with family members, and oversight of staff that were part of his daily work. He kept a dress shirt and a few ties in his office in case he was called to a meeting off site.

Mr. Hill's prior experience as a nursing home administrator influenced the way he operated Huntington Inn. He was used to the many federal regulations that govern nursing home operations and found the state oversight of the assisted living facility to be relatively light. He described his approach to running this family business as involving more interaction with residents than was the case in the nursing home. He said, "If I'm going to be the administrator I have to be accessible. This is not the nursing home level where they are basically bed bound and things like that. These people have a mind and are aware and I should be accessible. I think it has worked." We often saw him joking with residents, including Karen, and he was on a first-name basis with their families.

Karen and Mark agreed that Huntington Inn was a good fit with one exception—she could afford to live there for only about two years based on her limited income and savings. Before she moved in, Mr. Hill explained to Mark that the state had a Medicaid "waiver" program that paid for assisted living care and that he would help Karen apply for this program a few months before her money ran out. Unfortunately, this happened at the wrong time, when the state's allotment of Medicaid waiver resources had been exhausted by a large and unmet demand.

Karen was generally pragmatic and resourceful—she was one of the only women at Huntington Inn who did not have her hair "done" by the beautician who visited once a week, and she furnished her room with a "perfectly good" bureau found discarded by a trash dumpster near her son's home—and she spoke her mind and stood up for her rights. She believed in playing by the rules, but the changes in the Medicaid program, which she perceived as unfair, prompted her to action.

Getting to Know Huntington Inn

Overall, this assisted living was not a place that I liked to spend a lot of time, and I was always glad to leave. I found the physical environment depressing—everything seemed brown, the building was hidden in a wooded, rural location with no sidewalks. In addition, the staff members were never welcoming, though most were willing to answer my questions when asked. Most of the residents were friendly, but many of them had memory loss and did not recall who I was from week to week, even though I visited weekly for nearly 11 months.

A typical research visit to Huntington Inn would last for three to six hours. We learned to avoid the late afternoons because many of the residents were either napping or watching *Dr. Phil,* and no one wanted to turn off the television to talk if the doctor was holding court. Occasionally a group of three or four women took part in an event organized by an on-again off-again "activities director," but the most common activities we worked around to interview the people who lived at Huntington Inn were television watching, napping, dining, and medical appointments.

When you enter someone's home for the first time, you become aware of its differences from and similarities to the way that you live. There are different odors of food, pets, cleaning products, and various bodily functions. The meals that are prepared and served might look and taste different from what you are used to. The style and layout of the furnishings may not be to your liking. Our sense of Huntington Inn was that it reflected, not the cruise ship model of assisted living, but a freighter that carries the heavy load of cargo that no one else can, or will, accept. Mr. Hill told us that he was known by local health and social service providers for taking on "difficult cases," including individuals with chronic mental illness who presented challenging behaviors.

Mr. Hill purchased the building in 1988 from its prior owner after working as a licensed nursing home administrator in another state. For 12 years he operated Huntington Inn under the state's domiciliary care rules. In 2000, Mr. Hill, like Rani, Maria, and hundreds of other operators in the state, applied for the state's new assisted living licensure category.

Huntington Inn is located in a rural region where the primary industry is agriculture and a major tourist attraction is a museum of farming. The building sits on a gentle hillside, and because the gravel entry drive is at a higher elevation than the building, the dominant view on approach is of the brown metal Mansard-style roof edging. Nearby, though not visible from Huntington Inn, is a large reservoir used recreationally for fishing. A covered walkway shelters the front door, and often one or two staff members shared a smoke break here with a resident named Ron, who often sat outside quietly puffing on his pipe.

An interior sitting area at the front entry had been remodeled with upholstered furniture in floral prints and silk plants, but the pale pink paint did not disguise the concrete block walls. The furnishings in the dining room, as well as the bed frames, bureaus, and bedside tables provided in the resident rooms, might well have been there since 1972, when the building was constructed. For several months, a yellow mop bucket was positioned under a leak in the dining room ceiling. Throughout the building, the lower parts of the walls, as well as most doorways, were marred with black scuff marks from the many wheelchairs and walkers that had rubbed against them over the years. All in all, the physical environment was dowdy at best, though one enthusiastic staff member posted a monthly calendar on a hallway wall decorated with signs of the sea-son—brightly colored paper leaves in the fall, pink hearts for Valentine's Day, and green shamrocks for St. Patrick's Day.

Mr. Hill designated most of the rooms as single occupancy, explaining that people prefer a private room if they can afford it. Even though the facility was licensed for 60 beds, usually only 30 to 35 individuals resided there at one time, including a woman who stayed for single months of respite several times a year. Each resident room had a microwave oven and a small refrigerator, a closet, and a private half-bath with a sink and a toilet. The rooms' furnishings included a bed and bureau, and many residents brought personal items from home such as small collectibles, pictures, television sets, and in rare cases, large antique furniture. At least two residents, both with a lifelong diagnosis of mental illness, had spartan rooms, devoid of personal objects other than clothing. Because of the wooded area surrounding the building, some of the rooms were dark, and most had an institutional feel, reflective of the era in which the facility was built.

Huntington Inn was licensed to provide the highest level of care per-mitted by the state. However, Mr. Hill required that all residents be capa-ble of getting to the central dining room with minimal assistance, by which he meant that the resident should be able to respond to a verbal reminder or, at most, require a staff member to walk with. Residents who used wheelchairs were expected to propel themselves to the dining room. Mr. Hill gave two reasons for this rule: first, residents with limited mobil-ity were difficult for his staff to manage (i.e., the staff worried about get-ting back injuries while lifting or positioning residents), and second, mo-bility was required to use the shared, centrally located shower room, another vestige of the building's age, which was not disabled-accessible.

A small locked and alarmed "special care" unit was designated for individuals with dementia. This unit was in the basement along with the commercial laundry room and was accessed via an elevator operated with a key. The unit consisted of one hallway with six resident rooms, a small dining/television room, and a shower room. Only staff members and fam-ily visitors traveled between the two floors of Huntington Inn; residents from the lower unit went upstairs only on the rare occasions that they left Huntington Inn for a medical appointment or social event. Upstairs resi-dents did not go to the lower level at all.

Huntington Inn's physical structure predated design standards for disabled accessibility, so although each room had a bathroom, the bathrooms did not accommodate wheelchairs. The building had a fire safety sprinkler system, an impressive commercial kitchen, and a well-stocked pantry. The resident rooms did not have emergency response systems; if someone fell or needed assistance, the resident had to shout, bang on the side of a trash can to attract help (as one resident who fell in her bathroom told us she did), or phone the front desk.

A one-way public address system allowed Mr. Hill to make announcements and to track down staff members. While talking with a resident, we might be startled by the sudden intrusion of Mr. Hill's amplified voice saying, "Amber, please call the front office. Amber, please call the front office. Thank you." Another technological adaptation that Mr. Hill relied on heavily was a series of video cameras mounted in the hallways that monitored all exits. As he sat at his desk, taking phone calls from vendors, prospective clients, family members, and physicians, Mr. Hill was able to view five small television monitors that projected the scenes of residents, staff, and visitors moving through the hallways.

Mr. Hill, like managers in family-owned assisted living settings of similar size, wore many hats. He was a hands-on administrator who also performed tasks of a personal care assistant if necessary, a social worker (determining Medicaid eligibility, meeting with family members, planning discharges and placements in nursing homes), and a skilled laborer who did routine building maintenance. From his years of experience in long-term care, he was knowledgeable and politically active in that field (he had testified at state Senate hearings, and his own long-term care language had been used in state legislation), and he was highly responsive to his employees.

Mr. Hill's personal qualities had a positive effect on his employees, as was evident in a low staff turnover rate. According to him, nearly 90 percent of his staff had worked at Huntington Inn for more than five years, including three who had been there for 12 years. Several of the staff members were related by blood or marriage, and his assistant manager had literally grown up at the facility, beginning as a direct care worker when she was a teenager. Mr. Hill described his strategy for selecting good-quality staff: "I see how they walk by the residents. I see if they stop and say 'Hi' to them. I see if they are the sort of 'shun them' type and walk around them. I pick up a lot from that, and with my sixth sense, and I guess my years of experience helps quite a bit."

One Christmas his employees gave him a plaque engraved with "Number One Boss," and this, along with many certificates of recognition from local organizations, hung on his office wall. In his words, his employees liked working for him because "I try to listen to the people. I try to make it relaxing. I don't make it sterile where they have to wear whites [hospital or nursing home uniforms] and things like that. I try to have them come in, in street clothes—to sort of blend in. You can see—as the administrator I'm in jeans a lot—and that's because I'm also into toilets—when they stuff up—but overall, that's pretty much what I usually try to do."

Life at Huntington Inn

I enjoyed Karen and typically stopped by her room on my visits to Huntington Inn. . . . Karen always recalled me and would greet me with a cheerful, "Hello, doll" or "How's it goin', hon?" There were days, though, when Karen was sad or feeling poorly, a combination of physical pain, anxiety, and shortness of breath. On these days, her voice was flat and she might tell me that she wasn't up to company. Other times she might be napping or at one of several doctors' visits. I missed her on the days that she was not available to talk.

From Karen, we learned that life at Huntington Inn is bounded by rules, but that rules can be negotiated or broken; that declining health and finances are an ongoing concern; and that change is a constant dimension of life. Some changes can be anticipated and planned for, some happen out of the blue, and still others occur gradually.

Karen's room, decorated with American flags and ceramic sculptures of eagles, was located a little more than halfway down the long, dimly lit hallway from the dining room on the main floor. Though many residents kept the doors to their rooms closed, Karen chose to keep hers open, in part because it provided better ventilation for her oxygen compressor, and because she liked to see who was going by. She enjoyed company and often called out to passers-by.

Mr. Hill once described himself as a "live and let live" kind of guy.

Although it seemed to us that Huntington Inn was organized by rules, both internal and external, when one researcher asked Mr. Hill about his "house rules" he asked what the researcher meant, then said he didn't really have rules. Still, we learned about many expectations that rose to the level of rules during our fieldwork. These included the expectation that residents would wear street clothes (rather than bed clothes or a housecoat) to the dining room and that they would not use vulgar language. (Mr. Hill once admonished Karen for her liberal use of swear words.) In addition, all residents were required to receive assistance from a staff member to adjust the water temperature and get into and out of the shower in the communal shower room. Any residents who "wandered" had to move downstairs to the locked unit, medications for all residents were centrally stored and administered by the staff, and food from the dining room was not to be taken back to residents' rooms. Perhaps Mr. Hill didn't think of these as "rules" because he viewed them as practical necessities for operating an assisted living residence or because his nursing home experience led him to think of rules as externally imposed regulations. Over time, we learned that while there many "house rules," there were also exceptions to these rules.

Both Mr. Hill and the staff told residents that the assisted living regulations required all residents to receive assistance with a shower. The Maryland regulations for assisted living do not require this, though nursing home regulations do. (Most likely this small fib provided a convenient excuse to use with residents who complained.) Some of the residents openly resented this requirement, but Karen was pragmatic about it: "I feel as though I can do it myself. But then I'm just independent and I think I can do everything myself . . . but if I want to be really rational—I think I still need assistance." In contrast, Donnie, a woman of 69, complained that she did not like that a staff person entered the shower room with her—"but I can't do anything about it."

Despite this global requirement, two residents (one male, one female) were exempt; they each had a mental health diagnosis. It was difficult as an outside observer to discern the difference in physical functioning between Donnie, for example, and Ruth, the one woman who was permitted to shower on her own. When asked, staff members provided a range of reasons, including that Donnie "needed" help, that it was "required," that the water temperature was difficult to adjust, and that the shower stall was difficult to step into and out of, leading to concerns about a potential injury.

Another Huntington Inn house rule required that residents receive assistance with all medications and that the staff keep all medications in a central location. When some residents complained about this, they were told that it was a state rule. (Actually, state regulations permit assisted living residents to self-manage their medications if a physician indicates that the individual is capable of doing so. In such cases, residents must keep medications in a locked storage compartment in their own rooms.) Karen did not have a problem with the staff storing and administering medications because she took such a large number and type that she did not feel confident in managing them herself. Another resident, a retired nurse named Marge, described how she felt about the loss of control over her own medications: "Before you came in here, you had a brain, and you left your brain at the door when you arrived. And now your brain no longer functions. So that takes away independence on my part, you know, it makes me more dependent."

Another house rule prevented residents from taking food from the dining room back to their rooms, even though they had "kitchenettes" with a small refrigerator and a microwave. Again, the staff blamed this rule on state regulations, though no such provision exists. Residents were permitted to keep food brought in from outside the facility, but Mr. Hill required the staff to check that no perishable food had spoiled. The house-keeping staff regularly removed fruit they deemed as overly ripe—a practical strategy for preventing insects and rodents, but possibly an overly intrusive action into the "homes" of these residents.

Despite the strictness of dining room rules, there were circumstances in which residents were permitted to eat meals in their rooms. If someone was too sick to come to the dining room, it was possible to get a tray delivered from the kitchen (for no additional charge). Karen once complained that the staff "don't like to do it" because they don't want residents getting used to this kind of service. She said, "This is assisted living, so people should be able to go to the dining room."

Karen frequently ate meals comprised of food brought to her by her son because she did not like the food prepared in the Huntington Inn kitchen. She was especially offended by the way that food was presented—

"glop," according to her. When she had prepared meals, she had always made sure that the food looked good on the plate. Each day Karen would ask a staff member what kind of food was being served, and if she wasn't interested, she would say, "No, thanks!" or "I'm not coming" and would instead heat canned soup or stew. Mark made certain that his mother was stocked with canned foods, crackers, and soft drinks, and he occasionally brought a home-cooked meal or took her out for lunch.

For someone like Karen, who had worked hard at low-wage jobs her entire life, living at Huntington Inn felt almost glamorous: "It feels like home with servants. I can do what I want to in my room. It's just anything goes here." Some assisted living settings will not accept a person reliant on oxygen, but Karen, who was capable of managing it herself, presented no demands on the staff for extra attention. It is likely that if Karen had had any type of cognitive impairment, this arrangement would not have worked, either at Huntington Inn or at almost any other assisted living residence (Chapin and Dobbs-Kepper 2001).

Like many of the other residents, Karen used a walker or wheelchair to move around her room and the building. As already mentioned, Mr. Hill required that residents be capable of independently transferring to and from a wheelchair and that they get to the dining room without staff assistance other than the occasional verbal reminder. He described limited mobility as a "red flag" issue when determining whether to admit or retain a resident. Resident mobility was a major issue because of the staff: Huntington Inn had only a small number of direct care staff working each shift, and most of them raised concerns about heavy lifting that might result in back injury. In fact, several of them told Mr. Hill that they would quit if they had to lift heavy residents, and Mr. Hill agreed that it was more desirable to maintain his staff than to keep a resident, especially given the demand for affordably priced assisted living facilities like Huntington Inn.

We observed how one resident, Martha, declined over a period of several months. Technically she was capable of walking and transferring to and from a wheelchair, but she had fallen several times and, because of her weight and size, it took two to three staff members to lift her from the floor. The staff complained to Mr. Hill that Martha should leave, but he hesitated, instead suggesting physical therapy and weight loss. A complicating factor, however, was Martha's incontinence. Not only did she refuse to wear pads or briefs, but also she would urinate into containers rather than using the toilet, which, in her opinion, sat too low to use without extreme difficulty. She used empty food containers and plant buckets for this purpose and had spilled the contents onto the floor on more than one occasion. Her room and the hallway adjacent to it reeked of urine.

The staff, residents, and their families complained to Mr. Hill, yet he tried to make the situation work because he knew that no other assisted living facility would accept someone with Martha's complex problems. He asked Martha's son to intervene, and although the son tried, he could not change her behavior. Mr. Hill asked a geriatric psychiatrist who had a consultant relationship with Huntington Inn to evaluate Martha; the assessment suggested mild dementia and a possible personality disorder, but no solution. Finally, Mr. Hill asked Martha to move and helped her locate a small group home. He complained that the administrator of that home, a nurse, had immediately placed a catheter into Martha's bladder as a solution to her toileting behaviors. He did not believe it appropriate to use such a medical solution. The carpet in Martha's former room had to be replaced, and the concrete floor underneath had to be treated with an industrial cleaner. Still, it was weeks before the odor dissipated.

Despite having implemented a large set of house rules that were sporadically altered, Mr. Hill was well liked and respected by the majority of residents, their family members, and the staff. They found him to be helpful, supportive, and knowledgeable, especially about all matters bureaucratic. He knew how to work the system when it came to medical insurance, Medicaid, specialist referrals, nursing home placements, and hospital discharge, in part because of his community connections.

Community Connections

Mr. Hill maintained a professional relationship with the county aging services department, two regional hospitals, several physicians and related therapists, and two nursing homes. When a Huntington Inn resident had to go to a nursing home for postoperative care or rehabilitation, he would visit that individual in the nursing home to assess whether or not he or she would be able to return to the assisted living residence. As we describe in the following section, Karen's extensive medical ailments and treatments required collaboration between her, her son, multiple physicians and surgeons, Mr. Hill, the direct care staff at Huntington Inn, and both public and private insurance providers. Karen's son and Mr. Hill took the lead in managing the complex array of individuals, organizations, and regulations that overlapped in her medical care.

When compared to other assisted living providers, Mr. Hill had an unusual relationship with medical service providers. He not only arranged for a physician group and psychiatrist to make regular visits to see any resident who wanted in-home visits, but also coordinated with a lengthy list of mobile medical services such that, on a typical day, in addition to the regular staff, a physician, a physical therapist, a counselor, and/or a mobile X-ray technician might be on hand. These services were important in a rural location with limited public transportation. In addition, he assisted with Medicare billing. Several residents and their families mentioned these services as a reason that they appreciated Huntington Inn.

Changing Finances

Responding to a question at our first meeting, Mr. Hill said he accepted Medicaid payments on behalf of clients because serving lower-income individuals was part of his mission. He went on to explain that the Medicaid waiver program was new to the state and that there were many uncertainties about it, including whether the number of slots (i.e., individuals receiving a subsidy) in the program would be expanded to meet demand.[1] "The climate is not good to do the expansion of another 1,000 slots," he remarked. "We are hoping that they will expand to another 1,000 because . . . in the long run it has saved people from going into nursing homes prematurely because they didn't have the money to subsist in assisted living. . . . And also if they can subsist in assisted living, it is better for them. If they [the state] do not fill the additional 1,000 slots, then what's going to happen very quickly is there will be a waiting list . . . and I don't know what will happen at that point."

During our time at Huntington Inn, Karen's finances declined to the level that she qualified for Medicaid, but by the time this occurred, the "wait list situation" that Mr. Hill feared had occurred. When Karen ran out of money, the state's allotment of Medicaid waiver slots was full, so her only option was to go to a nursing home or attempt to locate a facility (most likely a small one) that would be willing to accept Supplemental

Security Income (SSI). She was used to modest means, saying that she was "born poor" and grew up in a "Baltimore ghetto." Three months before she would "spend down" (a bureaucratic phrase to describe the process of becoming financially impoverished enough to qualify for public subsidies) to the Medicaid-eligible income level, she said, "I'm a little bit worried because my money is running out and something about getting a—I don't know anything about this stuff; my son takes care of it—but something about getting a waiver and going on social services, and now they say they're not giving waivers. And I said, 'Well great, what happens to me now?' Now I got two things to worry me."

The second worry was a lump she had discovered in her right breast. Her doctor had examined the lump and recommended a mammogram. Mr. Hill arranged for a mobile mammography unit to come to Huntington Inn. Before receiving what turned out to be a diagnosis of cancer, Karen explained that she was more worried about where she would live than about having cancer: "I'm not worried about [the mammogram], because what's going to be is going to be. I have no control over that. God grant me serenity to accept the things I cannot change. But I do worry about where am I going to live? You know, that worries me, because I like it here. I don't know what's going to happen, but we'll see."

Karen had a strong sense of what is fair and right in the world, and after being told that the previously described waivers were not available, she said, "That's not fair; they take all your money and then tell you it can't be done. That's hittin' below the belt." Although she relied on her son and Mr. Hill to negotiate on her behalf, she took action by sending a letter explaining her case to the governor, a state senator, and the county aging services department. Staff from the county agency received and responded to this letter by meeting with Mr. Hill about how to address Karen's situation.

Mr. Hill arranged for Karen to enter a nursing home for one month and apply for a waiver slot from there. He worked with county agency staff to develop this plan because he knew that the state gave priority to nursing home residents who were capable of moving into assisted living facilities. Karen would need to stay in the nursing home for at least 30 days under this plan, but it was the best that could be done given the circumstances. Mr. Hill agreed to save her room for her, even though he would lose one or more months of rent. Karen's surgeon scheduled her mastectomy to occur during this time, so that her nursing home stay would coincide with the spend-down period.

Karen told several other residents and staff members about her change in finances and impending move out of Huntington Inn. Her friend Donnie told us, "I have this one friend in here—her name is Karen but she's leaving and she's going to a nursing home because she is running out of money. . . . She's upset, and I feel bad for her but there ain't nothing I can do. It might happen to me someday. This whole thing scares me. You know, you never know what your future is going to be."

During this time of financial uncertainty, both Karen and Mark speculated about possible alternatives to living at Huntington Inn. Karen hated paying $2,000 a month, and she wondered where else and how she might live outside of Huntington Inn. Mark considered renting a large apartment where Karen and two or three other women could live together, with him providing support in the form of groceries and transportation. Whether or not Karen "needed" assisted living was a constant topic of debate, but the question was answered to Karen and Mark's satisfaction by a county case manager who assessed Karen at Huntington Inn to determine whether she qualified for nursing home placement. Mark explained, "The lady that came in and evaluated her at the assisted living said there's no way she could live alone." Even though Karen had an independent spirit and could do many things for herself, she, like several other residents, experienced many declines in health, both acute and chronic, during her months at Huntington Inn.

Changing Health

Karen was in many ways like other Huntington Inn residents—female, a mother, Caucasian, and proudly blue collar. At 75, she was relatively young, but like the others she had multiple chronic health conditions, including a hip fracture in the month before she moved in, as well as emphysema, cancer, anxiety, clinical depression, and macular degeneration.

When she had moved into Huntington Inn a few months before we met her, she came directly from a nursing home, where she had received physical therapy following hip surgery. For the first year that she lived at Huntington Inn, Karen's health was stable, despite some minor illnesses and a bout of depression that was treated with medications and counseling. During her second year, she experienced several changes in her health that required hospitalizations, nursing home admissions, laboratory work, and multiple medication adjustments.

Karen entered Mt. Pleasant Nursing Center with the hope that her stay would last for 30 days, enough time for her to have the mastectomy, recover, and apply for the Medicaid waiver that would allow her to return to Huntington Inn. We visited on her second day at Mt. Pleasant and found her in good spirits. She was in a four-bed room, though one of the beds was vacant. As we visited, one of her roommates slept and the other one appeared to stare into space. When asked if the nursing home was different than she expected she said, "Yes. My mother-in-law was in a home and it smelled like urine. When Mark brought me in [here], and we came out of the elevator, there was no smell." She nodded her head toward one of her roommates and said, "She had a BM in bed, they came and changed her right away, and there was that smell, but they took care of it. It wasn't what I expected, far, far from it. This is a nice place. They should all be like this."

Karen said the staff had been wonderful ("They can't do enough for you"), that the food was excellent, and that the dietician had promised to bring her own Yorkshire terrier for a visit. During the hour that we visited, several staff members entered the room. One came in with an adult diaper in hand and closed the "privacy curtain" surrounding the roommate's bed, the unit manager asked if Karen's additional oxygen supplies had arrived (they had not), a maintenance person stopped by to fit an oxygen tank holder to her wheelchair, and a kitchen staff person came in to clear lunch trays. The hallway, visible from Karen's bed, was filled with medication carts, food carts, cleaning crews, and staff wearing a variety of uniforms. The public address system seemed to be in constant use to page employees and direct them to provide assistance in various resident rooms. Despite all of this activity, Karen said that she had slept well her first night, probably because of the antianxiety medication she requested and received. Asked if the lack of privacy bothered her, she said that in the nursing home, "modesty's ridiculous" because "what the hell, we're all in the same boat."

Karen returned to Huntington Inn after nearly five weeks at the nursing home. A couple of weeks after her return, she passed out, was transported to a hospital, and was diagnosed with a collapsed lung. She returned again to Huntington Inn, but after a few weeks had another collapse and acute disorientation when she didn't recognize others or where she was for several hours. After a week in the hospital she was sent to yet another nursing home, this time for physical therapy. Three other former Huntington Inn residents were also at this nursing home, called Meadow Hill Rehab Center. Once again, we visited to see how she was doing. Karen was not as positive about Meadow Hill as she had been about Mt. Pleasant, and she was anxious to return home to Huntington Inn. She told me that Mr. Hill had stopped by the day before and encouraged her to get stronger so that she could independently get from her room to the dining room. When we asked how she felt, she said that "the bridge has fallen out from under me" and that "if I stay here till I die, big friggin' deal." But she did not die; she returned to Huntington Inn after a seven-week stay. A short time later another member of our research team asked Karen whether Huntington Inn felt like home to her and she said, "Yes. I can mingle with my, the ones that live here with me, play games, and in warm weather we can go out to a beautiful patio. It's just anything goes here. The staff is just like your next-door neighbors. They're real friendly, you know. You kid with them. I really like it here. You can't compare this with the other [referring to a nursing home]." Although Karen had good days, her health continued to decline. Mark complained that she refused his offers to take her out to lunch, even to her favorite fast-food restaurants. Karen responded that she lacked both the strength and the will.

Over the months of fieldwork at Huntington Inn, we also witnessed health changes in several other residents. These changes included some improvements in physical and mental health, but more frequently change involved decline, both sudden and gradual. Living in a licensed setting like this one meant that health was an ongoing concern, a topic of conversation among all involved, including residents, family members, staff, and the various health and social service providers who routinely visited Huntington Inn.

Karen was a good source of information about health concerns, and not only her own. She was sociable and got her information from a variety of sources, including other residents, their family members, and the staff. During one conversation, she told us about the interactions that she and others in The Forum had with Ms. Frannie, a woman who had resided at

Huntington Inn for only two months: "She's also got a brain tumor. I guess it's inoperable. She got really bad. She'd come down the hall— sometimes she'd come down the hall, sit with us—she'd bring a box of candy and offer it to us. She was so nice. And when she'd get paranoid— she'd come down and she'd say somebody's out to get her. And we'd say, 'Sit down with us,' and she'd say, 'No, you're down here planning to kill me,' and we had a hell of a time trying to convince her no. And I felt so sorry for her. And she got real bad—so they put her down on first [the basement-level dementia care unit]."

About another resident, Karen explained that the woman would not return from the nursing home because "she's lost her will to live." Still another had had a stroke and could no longer walk. Philosophical at times, she explained, "Yeah, you see them come and you see them go. And you see them fail. You can watch them start to fail. Maria is starting to fail. She's fallen twice now in a month and—she come in the room the other day [acting oddly] and I thought, what in the hell's wrong with her?"

One of the more complicated cases involved "Mother," the woman with significant dementia who carried a doll. Mr. Hill wanted to move Mother to the basement unit because she attempted to leave Huntington Inn on a regular basis. One time she had walked about half a mile to a two-lane highway, where she had been picked up by a police officer. However, Mr. Hill's relocation plan was resisted by Mother's family and the direct care staff, who had known her for a long time and did not want to see her sent "down there." For an outsider this resistance was difficult to understand because the basement unit did not feel measurably different from the main floor, and Mother would have been prevented from wandering out of a locked unit, increasing her safety and diminishing the oversight required of the staff. A few of the residents complained about Mother because she entered their rooms and either refused to leave or tried to take their clothing or other personal items. Donnie, in particular, had no tolerance for Mother, and what started as rude nonverbal gestures between the two women eventually deteriorated to a physical brawl. Fortunately, neither woman was seriously injured. Donnie was furious because Mr. Hill defended Mother, even though that "crazy" woman had been in Donnie's room, but Mr. Hill countered that Donnie should be more understanding.

When we asked Mr. Hill how he determined when it was time for a resident to move to either the basement unit or a nursing home, he said, "I'm not trying to pat myself on the back—but because of my experience, I'm pretty good at telling when a person is beyond what we can do and needs a different level of care—for example, nursing home—so I'm pretty good with doing it on my own, but I do . . . I keep an open door policy with the families and if there is something to discuss, we will discuss it and so they pretty well know as their relative or loved one is slipping and getting to the point where, for the most part, they may need another level of care. My years of experience—and also my background in nursing homes—helps me to know the differences and what we can do and where we really have to draw the line."

The difference between nursing homes and assisted living homes is a topic familiar to anyone who has worked in long-term care. As Mr. Hill told us, and as we learn from the experience of Karen and other residents, there often comes a time when an individual requires nursing home care for financial or medical reasons. Sometimes the line between nursing homes and assisted living facilities is clear, but increasingly it is blurring. For example, Karen died at Huntington Inn under hospice care. In some views, end-of-life care might seem more like a nursing home function than one suitable for assisted living. In the final chapters of this book, we talk more about the complexities that arise in the larger world of senior housing.

Final Thoughts

Resident Changes

Residents came and went at Huntington Inn. One resident stayed only three days before the physician associated with Huntington Inn identified blood clots in her legs that required surgery; afterwards she did not recover sufficient strength to return. Another person went to a nursing home and stayed for several months, but contrary to everyone's expectations, she came back. There were changes (more negative than positive but of both kinds) in physical health, cognitive ability, and financial status. Sometimes a resident's family member initiated relocation, moving the relative to a place that was closer to home, less expensive, or perceived to be of better quality.

When we began our study at Huntington Inn in January 2003, there were 33 residents. During the next 11 months, 14 people moved out, 3 people changed rooms, 11 new people moved in, and 3 died. At a follow-up visit in 2006, we learned that 12 of the original group we met had since died. So the resident population is not stable over the long term, with both short-term interruptions for hospital and rehabilitation visits and regular turnover.

Regulations

The rules and regulations of assisted living, both those set by the facility and those mandated by the state, provided the subtext of life in Huntington Inn. Like Valley Glen and Franciscan House, this assisted living setting predated the state's regulations. Mr. Hill's prior experience in nursing home administration provided ballast as he rode the new wave of assisted living. When he began operating Huntington Inn, it was classified as a domiciliary care facility, a type of group residence that was not licensed by the state (although subject to various state and local rules and codes). Over time, Huntington Inn weathered changes in state regulations, public financing, new licensure categories, and competition from newer and prettier places.

Mr. Hill took an active role in two senior housing trade organizations and in policy workshops organized by a state agency. He explained that he wanted to represent the interests of the "folks" from his rural community—namely, low- to moderate-income individuals. He was articulate about the need to keep assisted living regulations flexible and to make certain that the state did not create regulations that would turn these settings into nursing facilities. In contrast to Mr. Hill's message, the public agency that licenses assisted living institutions in Maryland heard from senior advocates and medical professionals about the need for additional regulatory oversight.

One issue debated in a series of public policy forums was whether or not to require on-site licensed nursing staff. Mr. Hill regularly attended these meetings and argued against the need for on-site nursing at facilities like his; he explained that if he had to hire a nurse for 40 hours a week, he'd have to raise the fees for residents to $4,000 a month. People in his rural, agricultural community could not afford to pay much more than $2,000 a month, he argued. The assisted living facility located closest to Huntington Inn, a well-regarded dementia care facility, charged $6,000 a month, but attracted its clientele from the larger region because of its reputation. In addition, Mr. Hill said that he did not know what he would do with a nurse in his facility for 20 hours a week, much less 40 hours. He explained that there was just not that much for a nurse to do with 30–35 residents because the residents "don't change that often." He also knew that finding a licensed nurse in his rural region would be a major challenge.

Money Matters

As Karen introduces us to life in Huntington Inn, her story also provides lessons about what life is like for a woman of her cohort. Like many in her generation, she stayed home to raise her son and worked sporadically at low-wage jobs. As a result, she could not afford to pay for assisted living from her own resources for much more than one year. Over the course of less than a year, Karen spent down to the Medicaid-level income at the worst possible time: because of a cap no new Medicaid waiver slots were available from the Maryland Department of Health and Mental Hygiene, thereby limiting her access to care. Assisted living is frequently described as a consumer-driven model of care (Carder and Hernandez 2006; Kane and Wilson 2001). Karen's case reveals the limited and constrained "choices" available to low- to moderate-income seniors who cannot afford to pay monthly charges of $3,000 or more.

The lessons of Huntington Inn suggest that the story of assisted living centers on change. Through Karen's experiences, we saw changes based on declining physical and financial resources. As Karen told us, some of these policies are not "fair" to people who played by the rules during their lives. We learned about the importance of community connections among multiple parties, including the assisted living staff, the resident's family, public agency staff, social service and medical providers, and advocates. The rules and regulations of assisted living, both those set by the facility administrator and those mandated by the state's administrative rules, provided the subtext of life in Huntington Inn. The key theme of change became evident in the dynamic manner in which rules were negotiated between the residents, their families, staff, and various people and organizations outside the facility.

Update

Our primary fieldwork at Huntington Inn ended after 11 months, but through follow-up visits and telephone calls we learned of two significant changes. Mr. Hill died suddenly, leaving a gap that stunned the staff and many of the residents. (Some residents with cognitive impairment did not seem to notice or understand his absence.) The family hired a manager who made several unpopular changes; she was fired after a few months and replaced by a woman who had once worked in the county agency on aging—in fact, she had advocated on Karen's behalf after receiving Karen's letter many months before.

After more health problems and hospitalizations, Karen's doctor diagnosed her as terminally ill, due to a combination of cancer and COPD. She was placed under hospice care at Huntington Inn, with the hospice staff coming to her small apartment to provide comfort care. Karen died several weeks after her last return to Huntington Inn from a nursing home. One of the direct care staff members proudly reported to us that Karen had died "at home."

FIVE

Mrs. Koehler at Middlebury Manor

I don't know where else I would want to be. I really don't. I mean, there's a lot of big places around with big names, but that didn't interest me in the least. I would rather be right here. I really would, because to me it's just a family.

—MRS. PIERSON

Just in from sunning herself on the front porch, a tanned Mrs. Koehler confidently maneuvered her motorized wheelchair off the elevator and around the wheelchairs and walkers that crowded the hallway outside the hair salon. She cheerfully greeted everyone but did not pause to chat. The white noise and warmth from the portable hair dryers in the hallway had lulled some of the waiting ladies to sleep. Call-buttons buzzed, and James Taylor crooned over the intercom system. It was Wednesday, Jennifer's day to shampoo and set residents' hair. With what some might regard as "airs," Mrs. Koehler whirred past the smell of hair spray and the sleepy women, not wanting to miss the next rerun of *Law and Order*, the program around which she ordered her day.

Upstairs, in one of the recently vacated private rooms, Middlebury Manor's administrator was replacing light bulbs and cleaning the carpet. The activity coordinator was downstairs busily preparing for morning devotions and exercise class. An aide was wheeling the last of several residents from the dining room to the front sitting room, where the residents would sit quietly, only occasionally breaking the silence with a comment about the weather or the oft-repeated question "So, what is happening today?"

Middlebury Manor was the home of 81-year-old Mrs. Koehler and 40 other men and women. Through her experiences, we learn more about this place and what life is like for one of its residents. Like Middlebury

Manor, which has operated in the community for many years, Mrs. Koehler's social connections run deep. Her story illustrates the many twists and turns experienced by someone in later life as these events relate to long-term care, especially the movement between an assisted living facility and a nursing home, and reveals the personal emotions and cultural attitudes triggered by confrontation with hard choices. Her story also demonstrates the financial and interpersonal hardships families often encounter in this process. And we will learn more about the challenges small businesses like Middlebury Manor face in today's market and meet some of Mrs. Koehler's fellow residents.

Getting to Know Middlebury Manor

The Place and Its History

The unincorporated town of Middlebury borders a very large metropolitan city. Despite its proximity to a large urban center, Middlebury has an indisputable small-town feel. Middlebury Manor identifies itself as "low-cost provider," drawing most of its residents through word of mouth from this tightly knit middle-class community. It's not unusual for residents to have previously participated in a worship service at the Manor as a volunteer from the nearby church or to have paid a visit to a friend, neighbor, or relative who resided there. Residents tend to know each other or the family that owns and operates Middlebury Manor before moving in. Perhaps because of this, the residents of Middlebury Manor seem willing to accept occasional disruptions in facility services, even pitching in to help the staff with tasks of running the place when needed.

Middlebury Manor is a second-generation family-run and -operated assisted living facility. In the 1950s, Mr. Baker, the family's patriarch, purchased a poorly run board-and-care domiciliary home operating out of a turn-of-the-twentieth-century mansion. After some renovations and other improvements, he established a nursing home in the days before nursing homes were so highly regulated.

Nearly 40 years later, in 1992, faced with increasingly strict federal regulations, the next generation of the Baker family converted the mansion into an assisted living facility. It had become difficult to keep the building up to federal nursing home standards, so they decided to build a new 50-

bed nursing home connected to the original structure via an enclosed passageway. It made good sense to transform the mansion into a residence for assisted living, a model of care that was just taking off then and did not demand the same level of building and equipment requirements.

With a newly earned business degree and a nursing home administrator certificate in hand, Michael Baker, the youngest son, became the administrator of the newly formed facility, while his brother undertook the management of the nursing home. Given the family's experience in the skilled care business, their new assisted living facility adopted a more medical approach to care than some others, a contrast to the "social model" seen in so many purpose-built facilities. Michael's older sister, Carol, an RN with extensive nursing home experience, became the lead nurse. All of the direct care staff at the Manor were certified nursing assistants (CNAs), and the family hired a full-time licensed practical nurse (LPN), instituting practices that emphasized resident health and safety. For example, the facility LPN or RN conducts an in-house assessment when a resident has a complaint, as well as monthly weight checks and monitoring of all over-the-counter medications, in addition to the mandatory monitoring of prescribed medications—all services that are above and beyond state requirements. The Bakers chose to license the facility for level 2 care, a decision influenced by their skilled care experience. "We feel that if you're taking level 3 patients, you're acting as a skilled facility," said Michael. And with the nursing home next door, they anticipated a flow of declining residents moving from the Manor into the home.

Middlebury Manor represents a number of assisted living residences nationwide that are contiguous with a nursing home or part of a "continuing care retirement community," offering housing ranging from fully independent to assisted living and nursing home. In this case, the facilities are separately incorporated but share food services and some medical services, often shuttling residents back and forth. The Baker family sees movement between the two facilities as an almost seamless continuum of care. Residents, and especially their families, appreciate this continuity, reassured by the fact that the paired facilities are part of a small family business.

In 1998, the Bakers added a new three-level wing to the original mansion at the Manor, bringing the total assisted living capacity to 42 residents. The modest but comfortable rooms in the new wing all have chair-level floral borders, cream-colored walls, and private bathrooms and come with dark-wood Colonial-style furniture, now a little banged up and scratched from years of being moved in and out of the rooms. The entrance for the "existing building," as the original mansion is called by the family, opens into a large foyer with 10-foot ceilings, oak paneling, and a ceramic tile fireplace with carved oak columns flanking the mirror that hangs above the mantel.

Interior and exterior changes to the building over the years were influenced more by practical and financial considerations than by esthetics. It is sparsely decorated, with a single seasonally appropriate artificial flower arrangement adorning one of the several fireplace mantels. (Christmas time is the exception: strings of lights, music boxes, an artificial tree, garland swags, and wreaths are hung from every possible wall, corner, or shelf.) The wood floors are covered with short-pile industrial carpet, and the top of the once-open oak staircase has been blocked with a heavy metal fire door, detracting from the foyer's original beauty. Vinyl siding covers the exterior of both the mansion and the additions, with some effort made to tie the two together architecturally. The original front porch faces the adjoining nursing home and provides a roomy and comfortable place for residents to sit and watch people as they come and go. The residents share the front porch with the staff, who take occasional smoking breaks in one corner. Some of the space within the two-and-a-half-story mansion is used for administrative offices, as well as dining and activities; only 13 of the 40 resident rooms are located there.

The Residents

An African American hairdresser who comes to Middlebury Manor for the handful of African American residents there characterized the facility this way: Middlebury Manor gets "high ranks." By way of comparison, she spoke of an upscale corporate-chain assisted living facility in which she worked, the same chain that owns the Chesapeake (discussed in the next chapter): "That's the nicest of all. It's more for celebrities," she said, describing how many of the Chesapeake's residents are retired doctors, lawyers, judges, and other professionals. She said if you could afford it, the upscale facility is the place to be. But for "regular people, Middlebury Manor is really nice."

I grew to really enjoy visiting Middlebury Manor and the "regular people" I met there. As I did at the Chesapeake, I would play the piano for the residents. (The piano was purchased with the help of this research study's honorarium, replacing an almost-unplayable piano.) And I learned early on that, unlike many of the Chesapeake residents, who enjoyed Bach and Chopin, Middlebury Manor's residents generally much preferred familiar, popular music from the 1940s. Some would stick around after lunch to sing along as I played "Moon River" or "I'm in the Mood for Love." They taught me pinochle and offered advice as I neared the birth of my first child. I met family members, witnessed employees quitting or being fired, listened as residents complained and/or raved about the Manor, and attended several funeral services. My visits are much less frequent now and if I don't bring my children along, I'm good-humoredly scolded.

At one of our first visits to Middlebury Manor, we were invited to join a table of women for lunch. These women would be our entry point in this facility, greeting us warmly each time we visited. Mrs. Pierson wore a cluster of "pearl" earrings and a matching necklace. Nearly six feet tall, Mrs. Pierson was an imposing and yet extremely affable woman. She made a point of explaining how things operate in the facility. "They do our laundry and we don't have to cook our own meals," she said, although she noted that she brought with her to the dining room her own lettuce salad, which she kept in a little refrigerator in her room. She said the staff took them out shopping but would get anything for them that they needed. "They spoil us," Mrs. Hoffman said in response to this. "It doesn't spoil us," Mrs. Fitzsimmons replied. "Did you have someone doing all of that for you when you lived on your own?" Mrs. Hoffman challenged.

At our lunch, instead of the canned pear almost everyone else was served, Mrs. Pierson was brought a little bowl of red Jell-O. Mrs. Fitzsimmons said that every day, Mrs. Pierson ate her bowl of Jell-O. "I'm diabetic," Mrs. Pierson explained. Mrs. Pierson opened four individual-serving half-and-half containers and poured these over her Jell-O. After she was done, she opened up a little foil-wrapped loaf of zucchini nut bread she'd brought to the dining room and began cutting pieces to share. The bread came from a former neighbor of hers, she said. It wasn't sugar-free, so she wouldn't be able to eat any of it. She cut two pieces for the two ladies who sat at an adjacent table. One of the ladies, they intimated, was 103 years old. "Can you believe that?" Mrs. Pierson asked rhetorically.

These ladies would greet the residents as they walked, "walkered," or were pushed past their table. They seem to be the socialites of the facility. One woman noticed I was pregnant, and she told me she was expecting a grandchild soon. She said her 61-year-old son was having a child with his 33-year-old wife. And Mrs. Pierson proudly told me that she was soon to become a great-grandmother. She showed me the special individualized announcement of the pregnancy she received from her granddaughter. [Two and a half years later, I would finally meet her grand-daughter and her great-grandson at Mrs. Pierson's funeral.] After lunch I saw Carol [one of the administrators] again and I told her who I sat with at lunch. "Oh, the clique," she said with a smile.

Mrs. Koehler was not a part of this clique, instead choosing to sit by herself at a two-person table by the window. It was perhaps her "unhappy childhood" that contributed to her independent, self-sufficient streak. Her older sister had raised her after their mother was murdered. Her father, a house painter, was mostly absent. She never attended high school; instead, she started working as a telephone operator as a young teenager. When she had her own two daughters, she vowed to give them a better child-hood than she had experienced. She stayed at home full-time, planning scavenger hunts and outings to the park and the zoo. Their wooded back-yard was where all the neighborhood kids gathered to play. Mrs. Koehler, known for her scrumptious cheesecake and crab cakes, cheerfully enter-tained at a dining table that accommodated 24 guests.

Mrs. Koehler's Transition

When Mrs. Koehler and her husband entered their seventies, life began to change. Mr. Koehler, a retired vice president of finance at a local company, paid the ultimate price for his years of during-lunch, after-work, and evening cocktails. Diagnosed with cirrhosis of the liver, he suffered for nine long years with alcohol-induced dementia, unable to recognize even his wife before he died.

For as long as Mrs. Koehler's health and strength allowed, she cared for her husband in their home, changing his adult diapers and giving him baths. Her older daughter helped by arranging for the installation of a stair lift and checking in on them often. When Mrs. Koehler was unable to lift her husband from the floor after a fall, she would call 911 for assistance. Twice he fell on top of her. The operators at 911 finally told her that they couldn't continue to pick him up off of the floor.

Mr. Koehler's dementia had made it impossible for him to keep the bills paid and the checkbook balanced. His wife had never paid any attention to such matters and was not interested in learning. However, when Mrs. Koehler and her daughters were finally forced to examine the family finances, they were shocked to discover that he had mismanaged his money. The couple was tens of thousands of dollars in debt, with money still owed on a mortgage for the house they had bought 50 years earlier for $14,000. There were no savings. And yet for years the Koehlers belonged to the local country club, his position of social prominence earning him the moniker "Mayor of Middlebury."

Joyce, the older daughter and the self-described "doer" of the family, then assumed power of attorney for her parents. She spent the next couple of years navigating her way through the maze of elder law, Medicaid, and long-term care alternatives. She grew to know the long parade of Medicaid case workers by name. She filed and refiled for Medicaid eligibility for her father, amassing a huge amount of paperwork and becoming a fierce advocate for her parents. With this job as "paperwork person" came a growing resentment toward and disappointment with her sister, Anita. "I've talked to other people who were the paperwork person—they got pooped on and all the brothers and sisters get all the credit for the visits and the flowers and all the nice little things they do."

Anita was aware of the load her older sister carried and described their roles in this way: "My sister, Joyce, is the money lady, and I'm the . . . I drive Miss Daisy. I'm the emotional daughter, where I take care of all the necessities and visit and do all of the activities and get my mother out and about and run her to the doctor appointments. And my sister is a fantastic money manager, dealing with my mom. So we kind of split that responsibility. I say we both do what we do best. Because I wouldn't want to have that burden. Joyce has got a lot of burden on her shoulders." And ultimately, despite Joyce's frustration, she was grateful for the outings and appointments Anita took care of with their mother.

What the Koehler family was experiencing is common when adult siblings find themselves negotiating new roles as their parents become more dependent. More often than not, the greatest responsibility falls to the oldest child, usually the oldest daughter. And conflict of some sort often results. Specific tasks are (de facto or deliberately) assigned to particular siblings, often resulting in feelings of inequity (Matthews 2002).

Joyce continued to pour herself into the task of getting decent long-term care arranged and financed, motivated by a deep sense of loyalty and gratitude to her parents. Despite her efforts, her father spent the last years of his life in a substandard nursing home, with three residents to a room. She vowed to make better arrangements for her mother. With the help of an expensive but competent lawyer, she managed to do just that; the family held onto her father's life insurance policy, and her parents were able to keep their house. They benefited from the federal law known as the Spousal Impoverishment Law.[1]

Joyce and Anita sorted through their parents' belongings, donating and selling some, throwing out others. Joyce and her husband also made some needed renovations to the house after Mrs. Koehler moved into Middlebury Manor. "We've replastered, we've torn up carpet, we've thrown out stuff. There is no describing the process," Joyce said of the physical and emotional task of going through 50 years of stuff, her mother mostly unaware of the work that went on behind the scenes. Their hard work paid off. Like so many residents of long-term care today, Mrs. Koehler was able to reap the benefit of the coincidental real estate boom on the East Coast as the proceeds from the sale of her house helped fund her stay at Middlebury Manor.

Mrs. Koehler's Fall

Mrs. Koehler's move to Middlebury Manor, like those of so many assisted living residents, was precipitated by a fall in her home. Shortly before her husband died in the nursing home, Mrs. Koehler fell in her bedroom on the second floor of her home. This wasn't the first fall she'd had, but it became by far the worst. She landed uninjured on her bottom, but she was unable to pick herself up. She managed to scoot on her bottom to the stairwell, hoping for enough support from the stair lift to pull herself up. But she accidentally tangled her clothes in the lever on the chair, launching the stair lift down the stairs. Slowly and painfully, she was dragged down each step and deposited at the bottom of the stairs. It was almost midnight. She decided not to use the Life Line device she wore around her neck because she didn't want to wake anyone. Fortuitously, she landed near her recliner, where a crocheted afghan lay. She reached for the afghan, pulled it around her for warmth, and lay on the hard floor for the night. Her daughter said that her mother expected to die that night.

The next morning she awoke confused, unsure what had happened and where she was. The pain soon reminded her of the previous night's accident. She pushed the button on the Life Line. When she left her home by ambulance that morning, she would never return. No stranger to the Emergency Room, Joyce gathered her mother's necessary papers and medical records and met her mother and sister, Anita, at the hospital, prepared for a long wait and for bad news.

In this accident, Mrs. Koehler had severed all the ligaments and tendons in her leg and had broken six bones, including both shoulders. The orthopedic surgeon wasn't convinced Mrs. Koehler would make it through the surgery. He'd never seen her so despondent. He had patched up her brittle bones several times before, from hip to toe. He did her fourth and final knee replacement, her rotator cuffs, even a nose job. When he gave her the news about this latest injury, she folded her hands over her chest and closed her eyes. He actually took her pulse just to make sure she was still alive.

All her life Mrs. Koehler avoided doctors, but now that policy seemed to have caught up with her. She had broken her first knee replacement, brought on in part by her weight of about 250 pounds. The pain and subsequent surgery for a second knee replacement drove her to inactivity. She spent a lot of time on her recliner in front of the television with her feet elevated. So now, 20 years later, when she was dragged down the stairs during this most recent fall, she was "skeletally withered away," the orthopedic surgeon said.

She managed to pull through the extensive surgery, never to walk again. The surgeon wrapped a metal plate around her porous femur, saving her leg. Persistent anemia caused by deterioration of bone marrow made it necessary for her to go on weekly injections of a drug that built up her blood cells. She traded in her walker for a new motorized wheelchair paid for by Medicare. The wheelchair, it turns out, gave Mrs. Koehler the mobility and independence she had been missing. "It's a good friend," she once said of the chair.

Mrs. Koehler spent several months in rehabilitation at the nursing home run by the Baker family. Both she and her daughter lived about five minutes away, and the nursing facility was an obvious choice because they knew the Bakers. Mrs. Koehler had been a babysitter for the Baker children, and her daughter Anita dated the oldest son in high school.

Mrs. Koehler fully intended to return to her home after rehabilitation. She had no desire to stay in a nursing home and was anxious to recover. Living with one of her daughters was not an option she entertained. For years she had told her daughters: "Don't ever worry. I will never live with either one of you. Because I don't think it's fair. I have my own ideas and ways. It just doesn't work." For much of the Koehlers' married life, Mrs. Koehler's mother-in-law lived with them. "There is no house big enough for two women, believe me," Mrs. Koehler once said of those 30 years.

Eventually it became clear that Mrs. Koehler wouldn't be going home. Her doctors, her daughters, and the nursing home's administrator all agreed that she could not live alone. After several heated arguments in which her daughter told her that hiring a home care aide would be too expensive and that, further, no respectable agency would take on such a high risk anyway, Joyce said to her mother in frustration: "Go and fall to your death. You've said you want to die in your home. Go home." After some thought, Mrs. Koehler reluctantly agreed to the move: "I knew it was coming because my children wanted me somewhere so they could sleep at night, knowing that I was some place that someone would be aware of what was going on with me. And I realized that, but I still didn't want to do it. So that was really my deciding factor— to give my daughters peace."

The most logical next move was to the adjacent assisted living facility, Middlebury Manor. A couple of days before she was set to move, Mrs. Koehler drove her electric wheelchair across the covered passageway for a tour of what would become her new home. She felt more at ease when she met her soon-to-be roommate and admired the bright dining room, with its many windows and a gas fireplace.

Community Connections

Mrs. Koehler's room was to be on the second floor of the original mansion. Because of her limited finances, she would share a room with Mrs. Pierson. She immediately liked this woman, an affable lady with a commanding six-foot presence. Her name was familiar, and they soon discovered that their husbands had regularly played golf together. It turned out that Mrs. Koehler knew several residents in her new environment; she shared a hairdresser with one of the residents, and her daughters' grade school teacher had a room on the first floor.

Determined to make her move work, Mrs. Koehler put on a strong, cheerful front. In the beginning, she worked hard to adjust to daily life in this new setting, getting involved with the resident council, playing bingo and going on outings for lunch or shopping at Wal-Mart. Sharing a room proved to be a challenge, but she adapted to that change as well. The roommates would agree to watch the same programs on each of their televisions so that the sound of one would not compete with the other. One New Year's Eve, they invited a couple of residents to their room to bring in the new year. They served snacks and champagne and watched the ball drop in Times Square, along with millions of other Americans.

Middlebury Manor's Transitions

Adapting to Change

When Michael, the administrator of Middlebury Manor, started making plans to turn the second floor into a dementia care unit, he gave Mrs. Koehler the option of moving into a private room in the newer wing for the same rate she had been paying for a shared room. He needed to move the residents without dementia elsewhere so that he could add a dining room and eventually turn the few double rooms into single rooms. (Informed by experience, Michael had decided it would work best for each resident with dementia to have a single room.) He contracted with the local Alzheimer's Association to train his entire staff specifically for dementia care and worked directly with the staff to provide more individualized and dementia-specific activities for the residents of the "second floor," as the separate dementia care unit became known.

Until this time, residents with dementia had been intermingled with the other residents throughout the facility. Even with alarms on the doors and the front door pass code protected, on occasion a resident with dementia managed to slip out the front door and would later be found walking along the busy road bordering the property. Increasingly, some residents who did not have dementia had begun to complain about those with dementia, expressing disdain and annoyance at their behavior. A separate, locked unit would provide a safer environment and lessen these residents' annoyance; he also hoped the special services would attract more residents with dementia.

Mrs. Koehler immediately accepted Michael's offer for a private room, something she could not have afforded otherwise. She chose a room on the "terrace" level of the new wing, at the end of a hall, purposely away from a lot of traffic. She bought a new dorm-room-sized refrigerator to keep beer and other drinks cold for her visitors. Her daughter Joyce helped decorate her new room. Mrs. Koehler collected bird-themed items, and they hung her collection of cardinal decorative plates on the wall along with a shadow box of miniature birds; they also asked Mr. Baker if they could place a bird feeder outside her window. He agreed. Mrs. Koehler's nine-year-old granddaughter kept the feeder filled with bird seed. Joyce also placed flower boxes with colorful annuals near the bird feeder, creating a pleasant view from her mother's room. It wasn't until this move, one year into her stay, that Mrs. Koehler felt truly "settled in." Of her move to a private room she said, "I just adjusted [before]. But I adjusted more coming down here."

For Mrs. Koehler, life in assisted living was in many ways reminiscent of her life in the community. A "Lioness" with the local Lion's Club, she had volunteered for 30 years running the canteen at a local mental hospital. She stayed actively involved as a volunteer in her new home at the Manor. She took on the job of sending get-well, birthday, and sympathy cards to all of the residents and their family members. She was so efficient that at one point during our research she had birthday cards signed and ready for the next year. During one of the monthly Resident Council meetings, Michael Baker announced that Carrie, the well-liked activities coordinator, had decided to leave her job because Michael had had to cut her hours back. Mrs. Koehler cheerfully volunteered to fill in by arranging transportation for outings, funerals, and other outside events until a new coordinator was hired. Another resident volunteered to lead the exercise classes. The general mood during the Council meeting was positive, with several more residents willing to roll up their shirt sleeves and get to work, even though the activities they volunteered for were paid for by their monthly fees. Some residents, though, complained behind closed doors about Middlebury Manor's reductions in social activities.

Small Business Woes

Michael had been struggling to make ends meet with the doubling in liability insurance premiums, increases in health care costs for his employees, and increased staffing salary costs. The summer the second-floor dementia care unit opened was especially difficult. Several care staff members quit, forcing Michael to hire agency workers at much higher hourly rates. The occupancy rate at Middlebury had also been chronically low, a strain on a small business with an already-thin profit margin. More than 300 new assisted living beds had flooded the market nearby, dramatically increasing competition. Michael restructured the fee schedule to better reflect the costs of doing business. Instead of a flat fee for care, those residents who needed added care would pay more than those who didn't. For example, he instituted a "mobility" fee for those who routinely needed transporting to and from their rooms. He noted that the new fee structure "supplied us with the dollars to provide the services for the people who want to stay here, even though they do qualify for skilled nursing care."

The higher fees caught everyone off guard. A couple of residents revolted in a Resident Council meeting. "What is assisted living," one resident demanded, if it does not include assistance getting to and from the dining room? While the rates for some residents actually went down, for most the new rate structure meant an increase. Mrs. Koehler's rates went up 50 percent. Residents and family members complained bitterly. Joyce's response was outrage: "I could have understood 15 or 20 percent increase. I wouldn't have been happy with that either. But 50 percent! There's no way we could have prepared for this. What choice do we have [but to pay it]? We're selling her house, all of her furniture is gone . . . They know they have us. If we move her to another facility, we'll have to pay the initial community fee. And she's made friends here. It's also very convenient for us." (A community fee is a one-time entrance charge some assisted living residences assess as a way to cover costs for maintenance and upkeep of the building. At Middlebury Manor, the community fee in 2005 was $2,000 and was nonrefundable after 60 days.)

Although no one moved out because of the rate increases, Michael fielded many complaints, mostly from family members. Many residents, we discovered in our research, hand over their financial matters to family. One resident, a former accountant, noted the many empty rooms and fully recognized the facility's need to make a profit. But he, like the others, was most distressed by the cutback on activities from more than 40 hours per week to 20 hours per week and by the sudden departure of Carrie, the activities coordinator.

Employees' Concerns

Young and a bit hot-headed, Carrie had endeared herself to many of the residents by the way she corralled residents for morning exercise, her youthful energy stirring up what is often a sleepy, quiet place. And probably her most popular act, at least with the men, was serving ice-cold beer at the biweekly Men's Group she ran.

Carrie went out of her way by taking some of the more difficult residents under her wing. A good example of her enthusiasm for the "least of these" took place one morning during exercise. Miss Wry, one of the difficult-to-like residents, sat in her chair with her head propped up by her hand after being brought to the exercise circle by Carrie. As was usual, Miss Wry dozed in and out of awareness, completely unengaged. When the large, inflated ball would come to her, it would just hit her on the head and bounce off, and someone else would have to retrieve it. "She's sleeping," one resident commented. Miss Wry would half open her eyes but never look up. She didn't even take the initiative to kick it until, toward the end of the hour, the ball rolled to a stop right at her feet. She didn't stir. Carrie called out loudly, "Kick it, Miss Wry!" No response. Carrie didn't give up. She kept encouraging Miss Wry and the others began to join in. Finally, Miss Wry stirred enough to lift her foot and give the ball an anemic kick. The room erupted into cheers, and Miss Wry blithely resumed her semiconscious state.

Carrie showed special interest in Miss Wry, a woman with considerable cognitive impairment, precisely because she was difficult to engage. Miss Wry had no children or family. She was no staff member's favorite. Carrie's affection for Miss Wry and others like her seemed part of her sense of mission. Many residents were sad to see Carrie go.

Direct care staff had their own share of concerns. They complained about the many residents whom they labeled "nursing home material" that Mr. Baker, perhaps due to budgetary concerns, had started to accept and keep beyond the point they thought appropriate. These residents required extra care, and the direct care staff bore the brunt of that burden. For a variety of reasons, assisted living residences nationally, like nursing homes, are accepting sicker people than they had in the past. In the case of Middlebury Manor, the rationale was part philosophical and part financial. But perhaps a larger factor is the societal trend to remain in one's home as long as possible.

Mrs. Weston was one of the residents the direct care staff believed did not belong in assisted living. For as long as they could remember, she'd been unable to bear her own weight or roll over in her bed. It required two people or one well-trained person with a gait belt (a lifting and supporting device) to lift her. Some staff members had injured their backs lifting her. One staff member recounted the following incident with Gail, one of the direct care staff: "One day I heard somebody kept hollering, 'Help, Help'—so I walked back to Miss Weston's room. Miss Weston and Gail are on the floor. Miss Weston laid down alongside of Gail—Gail's on the bottom. Miss Weston done fell on top of her so many times—but this particular time they were in the middle of the bathroom floor. Gail on the bottom and Miss Weston right on top of her laughing. They say she still meets assisted living criteria. She can still feed herself. But physically, she can't do anything."

Some direct care staff members believed that Mrs. Weston was allowed to stay because she had been a resident for so long. Once when a move to the nursing home was suggested to Mrs. Weston, she cried and cried. "But I seen them get rid of people who was less work than her," one staff member said. Some more cynical direct care staff speculated that Mrs. Weston was staying because she was paying privately and was in no danger of running out of money. Ultimately, despite her physical impairments, Mrs. Weston was pleasant and generally liked by the direct care staff, another factor in determining who goes and who stays. Our research indicates that this is an example of the way that Middlebury Manor, like some of the other assisted living facilities profiled in this book, have rules but appear to enforce them selectively, based on a variety of complex and unpredictable factors. We discuss this issue further in Chapter 9.

Despite Mrs. Koehler's almost monthly cycle of going to the hospital and from there to the nursing home, she had always returned to her room in Middlebury Manor. Fluid built up in her chest and had to be suctioned periodically, a condition caused by congestive heart failure. Routinely, the care staff was forced to call 911 when Mrs. Koehler's breathing became too constricted. She good-humoredly dubbed herself "the comeback kid." But Mrs. Koehler's health needs put a strain on the care staff and greatly concerned Carol, the RN whose role it was to make all medical and health decisions. Carol did not feel comfortable leaving nonmedical care staff to handle a possible cardiac arrest or suffocation by fluid. When Mrs. Koehler was ready to return after one of these cycles, Carol determined Mrs. Koehler would need to move permanently to the nursing home. Mrs. Koehler's doctor didn't think she needed 24-hour nursing care, but the nursing home's physician disagreed. Mrs. Koehler told her daughter when she learned of this decision that she would die if she had to stay in the nursing home. At Middlebury Manor, however, Carol had made up her mind, and Michael initially deferred to his sister on this decision.

Joyce, Mrs. Koehler's older daughter and advocate, was well aware of the issues that stood between her mother's desire to stay at Middlebury Manor and Carol's unbending decision to not readmit her. While she understood Carol's fear of negative consequences should her mother die in Middlebury Manor, Joyce said she would never hold the facility responsible. She argued: "Why take away the private room, the cable TV? If she chokes to death on a crab cake, then at least she went out enjoying herself. My sister and I would rather she pass away in her room with a clicker in one hand and a Bavarian cream donut in the other."

Joyce described a move from Middlebury Manor to the adjacent nursing home as going from a luxury hotel to a budget motel. Her mother would lose so much. Lack of adequate space for a recliner would force her to stay in her motorized wheelchair or in her bed all day. And without cable TV service, unavailable in the nursing home, Mrs. Koehler wouldn't be able to watch her favorite show, *Law and Order*.

Despite Mrs. Koehler's complaints about Middlebury Manor's policy on restricting over-the-counter medication and what she reported as routine searches of her room for hidden medication, she knew that life in the nursing home would be even more restrictive. Ultimately, Mrs. Koehler was happy living at Middlebury Manor and did not want to move. She was content to let her daughter Joyce work on her behalf, pleading to her daughter not to let this happen but stepping back almost passively from dealing directly with Michael or Carol to wait for news of her fate.

Joyce frantically began to look for alternatives. She called several assisted living facilities in the area. She was upfront with them about her mother's health issues, with the consequence that many of these facilities refused to accept Mrs. Koehler as a resident. The one that agreed to take her later changed its decision when its staff came out to perform an in-person assessment. The stress and hard work over the prior four and a half years had taken a toll on Joyce and her family. "This is taking over my life, and it shouldn't," she said. "My kids have eaten pizza and cheesy bread and McDonald's, because I didn't have time. 'Oh, well, just get them a Happy Meal. I've got to get this done.'" Friends told her she looked like she had aged 10 years. She even permanently lost her hearing in one ear, caused by a virus brought on by stress, according to her doctor. But she felt she owed it to her mother to continue fighting for the best possible living situation. She loved her mother and wanted her to be happy, just as her mother had provided a happy childhood for her and her sister. She said, "You do it in honor of what your parents did for you as a parent."

After a few tearful conversations with Michael and Carol Baker, Joyce was suddenly told of an unexplained approval for her mother to return. Behind closed doors, Michael apparently overrode Carol's decision. The reason for this change was unclear: perhaps it was part of his plan to save money. He wanted to change Middlebury's medical approach to care to one that was "more assisted living," as he described his plan. In this case, he would consider making exceptions to allow residents to age in place, even if it meant making some compromises. Carol's nursing home background, in this case, might have been a barrier to moving in the direction Michael decided to take the facility to stay solvent. He had already eliminated the full-time LPN position and wanted to hire a part-time nurse with experience specifically in assisted living. If money was no object, he preferred the more medically cautious route. He once said, "My definition of a successful [transition] is 'appropriate'—appropriate for their safety, which typically involves making sure that they're receiving the proper supervision, monitoring and assistance that they might need." But in this case, he believed that keeping Mrs. Koehler was within state regulation. Joyce believed that her family's ties with the Baker family ultimately saved her mother from the move to the nursing home.

Middlebury Manor: Moving to a More Clearly Defined Assisted Living Paradigm

Michael had a record of being a flexible administrator, willing to accommodate financial shortfalls to allow residents to stay. "I don't think we'd still be here if we weren't. I mean we just don't have, we're not able to attract, the clientele that have enough money." This was welcome news to many residents and family members. And it also served the facility well by keeping beds filled. He liked to distinguish himself from the competition, noting that he didn't just "kick people out." For example, with doctor's approval, the Manor allowed one resident's son to come into the facility three times a week to bandage and clean his father's foot as a cost savings. And Michael started a subsidy program, allowing residents who qualify for Medicaid to move to one of the smaller rooms with no private bath, even though the state Medicaid waiting list was nearly 6,000 people long, according to Michael. The residents had to be able to pay at least the Medicaid waiver amount of $1,634 (2005 figures) to qualify for the Manor's subsidy. But if there were no small rooms available, the resident whose resources ran out might have to leave Middlebury Manor. Michael remarked: "You know, it's been challenging. But it works. People don't have to leave, and it keeps the families from having to mortgage their house to pay the bills or bring Mom home."

Michael came to realize that the higher fees he'd instituted in the previous year of our research there no longer made Middlebury Manor a good buy relative to the nearby competition, and perhaps was contributing to the lower occupancy rate. Again for financial reasons, he decided to essentially shift the way the Manor did business further from a nursing home model. "I made the mistake of providing all of these services, and before you know it, you realize you're providing a lot of services you aren't charging for. It's kind of a tug of war because the clinical is always at odds with the financial and the business side."

One of the benefits of being essentially a mom-and-pop business is the ability to receive direct feedback and change course as needed. In the end, Michael made some hard decisions to reduce some services (like social activities) and do some staff restructuring, allowing him to lower rates. Mrs. Koehler's rates decreased, but no refunds were given. A refund was never offered or considered because it was not even possible. "After going through 2003 and 2004, we kind of snowballed into this higher acuity level of service. Fact is people can't afford [the higher level of services and care]. And I've learned that, the hard way. And the people have exhausted their funds."

Mrs. Koehler's old roommate, Mrs. Pierson, suddenly found herself in this very situation. Unaware of her financial standing or of her son's monthly contribution, she was informed by her son one day that she was about to run out of money. Although she would have been willing to trade her private room with bath for one of the small low-cost rooms, none was available at the time. Moving to a smaller room in the Manor wasn't an option anyway, since her monthly income was too little even to have qualified her for the in-house subsidy. Tearfully she accepted her fate; she would be moving next door to the nursing home. She qualified for skilled care and could receive Medicaid funding there. Though in reality she was only moving next door, for her the move might as well have been across town. At first she held onto the hope of moving back to Middlebury Manor, but eventually she resigned herself to her shared room at the nursing home. As time went on, she rarely walked the short distance to Middlebury Manor to visit, stating that she was afraid of falling. Her entire social network had changed. Her living space had been reduced yet again, this time to two drawers and half of a small wardrobe.

Despite Mrs. Pierson's disappointment, she approached this transition in much the same way as she did her move from her own home to Middlebury Manor four years before: "You wonder how you can, you know, go through all that and it's just a loss of so much. But you learn to cope and you have to do it. I mean, otherwise you'd go crazy. You have to learn that—say, well, this is it. This is the way it's going to be, and you learn to do that. It's hard but you learn. And you can always look around and see somebody worse off than yourself. Absolutely."

Mrs. Jackson was more fortunate. A retired teacher with a decent monthly income, she could afford to stay in the facility provided she moved from her private room with bath to one of the smaller Medicaid rooms. Her son had been communicating with Michael Baker for the past year to plan for the imminent shortfall after her savings were depleted. And so, when the time came, Michael offered them the in-house subsidy, cutting her fees by about $1,000. The Medicaid room was about half the size of her first room, with no closet or bathroom. Mrs. Jackson now had a little sink in the corner and a tall but narrow wardrobe that served as a closet. "My son said I didn't need all those clothes anyway," she said with a laugh. She was remarkably positive about the loss of space and privacy: "Well, as long as I have a place to sleep and eat, I'm okay. I've lived a good life." She was grateful that Michael was willing to accept a reduced rate and that she was not forced to move. She wondered if he made this exception in part because she was one of the very few African American residents at Middlebury Manor.

Fortunately for Mrs. Koehler, running out of money was not a pending threat. Once back in her room at the Manor after her latest nursing home stay, she celebrated with her daughters by sharing a bottle of champagne.

Mrs. Koehler's health continued much the same way as it had: a buildup of fluid forced her to take oxygen and eventually led to 911 calls, a hospital stay, the nursing home for rehab, and then back to Middlebury Manor again. Each time, she came back a bit weaker. She then lost her ability to speak. Her throat had been persistently sore; to soothe it, she drank ginger ale, Sprite, and tea, all thin liquids. But this made her condition much worse. She'd been irritating her throat and literally aspirating the liquids. Over time, this damaged her vocal cords, all a part of her congestive heart failure and the buildup of fluids in her chest. Mrs. Koehler seemed resigned to this latest development, choosing to ignore the exercises prescribed or the order to eat only pureed food.

Her daughters were sympathetic to their mother's decision. Mrs. Koehler just shrugged her shoulders when asked about the exercises. Joyce said, "It's as if she's saying, 'It's just one more burden to carry.'" She couldn't imagine forcing her mother to live out her final days eating food that looks like "vomit," as Joyce described it.

Middlebury Manor continued to care for Mrs. Koehler despite Carol's persistent concerns and Mrs. Koehler's steady decline. According to Joyce, Michael was more understanding and became an advocate for her mother to stay there. And Mrs. Koehler was convinced that Carol simply didn't like her. She learned not to complain too loudly or to make too many requests. Like some other residents living in assisted living, she feared retribution by the direct care staff and administrators, the people she relied on for the most basic care and those who had the power to take away her home at any time. Warranted or not, this concern was echoed by others here and at other assisted living residences we visited.

Toward the end of Mrs. Koehler's life she developed a friendship with one of the long-time care staff members, Kira. Kira shared Mrs. Koehler's love for shopping, and one day when Mrs. Koehler's younger daughter, Anita, came by to visit her mother, the three started talking about a favorite new grocery store north of the city. Mrs. Koehler had never been there, and so Kira volunteered to go with them during her time off. Mrs. Koehler's daughter drove.

Kira smiled as she remembered Mrs. Koehler's reaction to the enormous store: "She liked to die and go to heaven." Mrs. Koehler spent more than $100 that day. And the experience cemented a friendship of sorts. Kira continued to accompany Mrs. Koehler and Anita on outings. When asked why she did it, she said she "went along just as a friend," not expecting or asking for anything in return. "We became real close" towards the end of Mrs. Koehler's life, Kira said.

Final Thoughts

When the Baker family first opened Middlebury Manor in 1992, Michael's father predicted assisted living would go the way of nursing homes and become highly regulated. He had lived through this very process with the nursing home he started in the 1950s. Assisted living had seen little regulation, but that is changing. "We're going down the same road now," Michael said of the recent state regulations and the ongoing discussion of how to implement them. "And it's not necessary to reinvent the wheel." Michael expressed annoyance when he heard that state policymakers and advocates were discussing the possibility of requiring all assisted living facilities, regardless of their level-of-care categorization, to keep an LPN on staff. Although Middlebury Manor had employed a full-time LPN in the past, he now found it impossible to support such a position financially. Michael recognized the need for an LPN for assisted living facilities that are licensed for level 3 but did not regard this as necessary for level 2 facilities, the level of Middlebury Manor. "Assisted living should stay light-skilled care," he said. He saw the proposed regulation as an "unfunded mandate." Out of frustration he commented, "If things continue as they are, I'll have to hire only agency people," unable to afford a regular staff and their benefits. "They'll come to work and I'll hand them a list of things to do: 'Four showers on this floor, etc.'" Michael was disturbed by a move in this direction and the diminished quality he foresaw arising from it.

As he noted: "Residents are coming into [the facility] more needy. In 1992, most everyone was ambulatory and needed more modest medical assistance." This trend is not unique to Middlebury Manor but is instead in part due to a larger national trend to age in place. Seniors are staying home as long as possible with the help of family or home health aides, or through sheer resolve. Once in assisted living, residents, with the help of their families, find ways to stay there, perhaps hiring a personal aide or accepting certain risks, negotiated between the administrators, families, and resident. Residents and their families, Michael noted, resist a move from assisted living to a nursing home, which carries an inescapable stigma. "When an issue arises, or you can even say in some cases, conflict arises because of transfers—typically if we recommend a transfer to [the adjacent nursing home] or another skilled facility, the resident and their family many times will not agree with that. They want to keep their private room; they want to keep the situation they have here. So we have to really draw a line in what we're able to do safely in-house with the staff that we have on our payroll."

Mrs. Koehler found herself in the middle of this very "conflict," to use Michael's word. Her highest priority had become avoidance of a permanent move to a nursing home. For her, transition was almost a constant possibility, so much so that it had become routine. When Mrs. Koehler cycled in and out of the nursing home for rehab, she understood the stay as temporary. But when faced with a potentially permanent move, she became fearful and full of dread.

Despite Michael's adamancy, as we learned from Vivian Koehler's story, the line is often drawn in the sand. For Mrs. Koehler, her declining health, the opinion of the nurse, the medical "culture" of the Manor, the facility's financial challenges, her daughter's tireless advocacy, and perhaps their personal ties to the Bakers all played a part in what transpired.

Update

Mrs. Koehler eventually succumbed to one of her many ailments, the drug-resistant staph infection MRSA that she'd contracted during one of her many hospitalizations. In the weeks before her death, a feeding tube was recommended, to which Mrs. Koehler replied: "Hell, no, I don't want to be on a feeding tube." And, despite the warnings of possibly choking to death, she brazenly took a swallow of the cold Classic Coke her daughters reluctantly gave her. "That tastes so good," Mrs. Koehler whispered.

A homecoming party welcomed Mrs. Koehler when she returned to the Manor for the last time. A banner made by residents hung on the door, and a small group gathered to celebrate her return. But Mrs. Koehler was tired and growing more and more weary. "She was worn out," Joyce said. "We were worn out." When the MRSA infection flared for the final time, Middlebury Manor called an ambulance, and Mrs. Koehler lost consciousness before her daughters arrived at the hospital. Joyce said that she and Anita kept watch for two days and were beside their mother as she peacefully "sputtered to a stop."

SIX

✿ Dr. Catherine at the Chesapeake

I met Dr. Catherine on my first morning at the Chesapeake. Standing in the lobby, establishing my bearings, I found myself in the middle of two lines of traffic, one group of women heading back to their rooms after breakfast, another group lining up to place lunch orders for the day's outing to a nearby restaurant. Within moments I was enveloped by a long leash, soon to be licked by a friendly white terrier. Bending down to pet the dog, I could hear conflicting comments from residents, ranging from one woman's exasperation about losing her balance to a "Good morning, Muffin" from an obvious dog-lover. I looked up to greet Muffin's owner, but my eyes met only the long leash. I made out its circuitous path, weaving through the legs of residents and walkers, ending in the hand of a petite, well-dressed woman talking to the receptionist. I soon learned that Dr. Catherine is a visible and independent, poised, rarely demure resident.

Dr. Catherine looks quintessentially Chesapeake. She dresses impeccably in periwinkle blue or azalea pink; the Chesapeake's decor is coordinated in patterns of hunter green and burgundy. She redecorated her suite several months after moving in, while the Chesapeake refurbishes at any hint of wear. Dr. Catherine purchased a new bed and vanity, and the Chesapeake ordered a pool table and baby grand. Though younger than most of her peers (in her early seventies), she mirrors assisted living residents in that she has been diagnosed with dementia, arrived as a result of a catastrophic event, and transitioned from her home into the Chesapeake through several medical facilities.

Over the three and a half years in which we got to know Dr. Catherine, we found her to be a sociable resident who walked her dog often, was active at residents' meetings, embraced the cause of smokers' rights, formed friendships, advocated for residents, and championed the basic assisted living values of independence and autonomy. In this chapter we follow Dr. Catherine through a dual transition, first one into assisted living and eventually a second into the dementia care unit. We discuss issues of entry and acceptance of an assisted living community as home; delve into the dynamic social relationships among residents, families, and staff; explore the role oversight plays in lifestyle change; and provide insights into the residents' perspectives on the values of assisted living and the administrators' balance of risk and comfort for all stakeholders at the Chesapeake.

Introducing Dr. Catherine

Dr. Catherine led an active life as an educator. She rose from classroom teacher to area supervisor, consulted in Africa and Asia, and earned a graduate degree while raising two children. Following her retirement, Dr. Catherine did nothing. Her friends, all teachers, were younger and still busy in the classroom. After a car accident, she gave up driving, thus restricting her movements even more. Her daughter, Susan, noticed that she was becoming increasingly disoriented, having falls and strokelike symptoms requiring hospitalization, and drinking after having been sober for 25 years. Her friends heard less and less frequently from her. Inadvertently, Susan discovered that her mother had been unable to learn how to operate the telephone answering machine. Her friends interpreted the lack of contact as lack of interest, when, in fact, Dr. Catherine was cognitively unable to respond.

Need for Assisted Living

Susan began to look for residential placements with graduated levels of care soon after she realized that her mother was having problems, but Dr. Catherine did not feel she was ready to move out of her home. Susan placed her mother's name on a list at one assisted living facility in the event that an apartment would be needed quickly. Dr. Catherine permitted this but would not visit the home nor meet with the elder care consultant Susan hired. Divorced and independent, Dr. Catherine on her own found a woman to help her. Susan did not approve of this person, as she smoked and drank. An MRI after a fall showed that Dr. Catherine's brain was "shrinking," and the physician spoke to both of them about alcohol-related dementia. Although this had been mentioned three years earlier, this time it "sank in," and Susan believed that her mother stopped drinking.

Several months later, Susan found her mother in crisis. She had had a "bad fall at her home. And you know, it was in between when people were coming to visit her. . . . We think she was on the floor for three days. . . . She has a very good friend. . . . They would call each other every day. He'd been calling and calling and couldn't get her, so he finally called the police and they found her. They were able to break in and they found her on the floor."

While in the hospital, doctors told Susan that her mother had severe Alzheimer's disease, but Susan and then later the Chesapeake staff never agreed with this diagnosis. Susan commented that her mother "had been on the floor with no food or water for at least three days" and feels this was sufficient cause for her mother's unsteady mental state. Dr. Catherine spent two weeks in the hospital and several more in rehabilitation while Susan combed through lists of assisted living homes.

Susan had six criteria for selecting a residence for her mother: safety, comfort, a social network, meals, dispensing of medication, and a home that was well kept and handsomely decorated. She had already reserved one room when a friend suggested the Chesapeake. The distance to her own home was longer, but the travel time was comparable, and Dr. Catherine's close graduate school friend lived only minutes away. The initial visit was positive, and Susan especially appreciated the grounds where her mother could safely walk Muffin. The Chesapeake had one opening, and Susan followed her instinct to switch homes. Although for months Dr. Catherine did not feel she belonged in an assisted living home and fought with her son and daughter not to stay, she still thought the Chesapeake "a pretty place."

Assisted Living as Home

Clare, the Chesapeake's assistant executive director, has much experience counseling families and residents, holds a graduate degree in gerontology, interned in and reorganized other assisted living homes, and ran the dementia care unit at the Chesapeake before her promotion to director of the assisted living wing. She advises family members to consider residents' feelings when they are moving in and to make their apartments as "homey" as possible.

Once acclimated to the Chesapeake, Dr. Catherine and her daughter together began to realistically define the comforts of "home." Dr. Catherine's rooms were on the first floor, an easy stroll to—or retreat from—everywhere: dining room, porch, elevator, television lounge, smoking area, and the outdoors with Muffin. Initially, her two-room suite was configured with the bedroom facing the parking lot and the living room opening to the corridor. The disabled-accessible bathroom and a closet are recessed and situated between the rooms, and a wide hallway allows light from the windows to filter through the apartment.

In the redecoration, Susan and her mother decided to switch the layout, and the couch, newly bought to fit the space, rested between windows to allow Dr. Catherine natural light for daytime reading. The double bed was exchanged for a small twin, placed along the wall in the inner room where the light is diminished and Dr. Catherine could comfortably nap in the afternoon. A large television sustained her penchant for national news, and a white portable television atop a bureau served for viewing during occasional insomnia. Dr. Catherine's diploma, sketches, and photographs were hung, and the bureau drawers marked with colors and clothing items so she could easily find what she needed. Dr. Catherine placed Muffin's bed, rug, and water bowl conveniently near the door, and she decided to retain her children's infant cradle to hold magazines and photo albums. Both women were pleased with the result of their decorating; it was something fun they did together.

Clare is realistic when it comes to understanding residents' frames of mind when moving in. "It doesn't happen very often that residents are coming in here like—'Oh, this is going to be great—I can't wait to move into the Chesapeake and leave my home of 50 years!' Usually they are very resistant to the move." Clare feels that eventually about 70 percent of residents call the Chesapeake "home." Gina, a care aide in her fifties and a favorite among the residents, empathizes with those under her care and tries to put herself "in their shoes." She commented that it "must be hard to leave your home of 40 or 50 years" and finds that residents often arrive angry and retreat for days into their rooms. Eventually, "they come around," and she hears, "It's really not so bad here!" as residents begin to participate in social activities.

Keeping Busy

The corporation that owns the Chesapeake prides itself on developing and offering distinctive activities believed to engage residents mentally and physically. Because Tammy, the Chesapeake's activities director, is intense about her work, she is treasured by some residents while alienating others. Dr. Catherine found Tammy's high-pitched voice and ageist and aggressive speech annoying because "She doesn't stop to listen . . . you know, she's always 'Come on Catherine, let's do this,' 'Come on Catherine, let's go do that,' and I say, 'Listen, listen—I have some reading I want to do.' She has always got something for you to go to. Well, I'm not a go-to person all the time. I can be by myself."

Structured activities did not initiate Dr. Catherine into the Chesapeake, but having a dog and being a smoker did. Muffin needed to be exercised, and while the Chesapeake welcomes animals, it is the responsibility of the pet owners to maintain their care. Muffin drew Dr. Catherine outside for walks, and the friendly terrier attracted other dog lovers. Dr. Catherine told me that she "would not have come" to the Chesapeake without Muffin.

Smokers meet in their segregated areas. Because cigarettes are not permitted in suites, Dr. Catherine requested cigarettes two or three at a time from the receptionist and smoked in the "smoking room," its location requiring a walk through most of the downstairs, or outside in the front of the building, where benches and a receptacle for cigarette butts are placed. Dr. Catherine got to know Dr. Smith in the smoking lounge, and through their repeated interaction, they developed a friendship. According to Dr. Smith, gender, age, class, and addiction formed the basis of their relationship. He astutely noticed that both he and a male dentist were always addressed as "doctor," but Dr. Catherine was often called by her first name. He spoke about her: "I think we have the same kinds of backgrounds. In the first place we're younger than—I mean the typical resident here is well into *her* eighties. I think there are half a dozen guys in the whole complex, the rest are widows . . . [and] well, we both smoke cigarettes, which I guess is a—probably not a very positive thing to have to admit to. But we enjoy each other's company. Put it that way. "

Throughout the many months of our research period, Dr. Catherine welcomed my visits. Most times she was happy to talk, open to discussion on whatever was headlined on CNN. There were times she was sleepy, angry, sad, or uncomfortable with leg pain. During the first year I was there, she was eager to implement a program bringing together residents in assisted living and the dementia care unit, and we brainstormed on how to put her plan into practice. Our visits were more casual than formal. One afternoon, as we sat near the window, Muffin on my lap, Dr. Catherine shared about her relationship with Mr. Peters, a "romantically interested" man who lived on the second floor. Other times Dr. Catherine and I met up outside or in one of the lounges. Dr. Catherine was not one to be holed up in her room, but also not one to be engaged in some planned activity. I learned to tolerate the smoking lounge as a good place to observe conversation between residents and an occasional well-liked staff member, especially on cold days when it was too uncomfortable for an employee to stand outside the kitchen door and smoke.

There was a period of time at the Chesapeake when two researchers were present, often on the same day. We put in days ranging from two to ten hours, attending staff, director, resident council, and food committee meetings; participating in and directing activities both in assisted living and the dementia care unit; learning who does and does not watch *Oprah* and *Dr. Phil;* chatting about local happenings while sitting on the porch; escorting a resident shopping or to lunch; and visiting with and interviewing residents and staff in suites and public spaces.

At the Chesapeake, the direct care staff assist residents throughout their shifts, and this includes most dining room duties, except for cooking and washing dishes. We "worked lunch" and occasionally helped at dinner, pouring coffee so the staff could take lunch orders, start the soup cart, and retrieve tardy or forgetful residents. Eventually we graduated to serving all beverages, learning who drinks what and how much and who groans at tepid coffee and confesses to caffeine jitters. We brewed coffee, served meals, set place settings, dished up ice cream, bussed tables, and changed soiled tablecloths. After lunch, several of us would sit around and talk about our kids, vacations, the residents, irritations, and the work of assisted living. In this way, we learned about and thanked an overworked and underpaid staff.

Lunch also gave insights into resident and staff interactions and conversations in a formalized group setting to which everyone—all but the sickest of residents—had to go or be charged handsomely for room service. One afternoon Mrs. Murtha, the most crotchety of residents, called me over to a seat in the café. Could I please apply her eyebrow pencil, she entreated, as she wanted to cover a bruise she received after her last fall. Try as I might, I couldn't raise a color. Much to my dismay, I noticed that I was applying a standard number 2 pencil! She accepted my apology, scrounged around, and finally found her Maybelline at the bottom of her walker bag. Pencil and lipstick finally applied, she stood up, adjusted her overshirt, and stately walked into the lobby, ready to face all.

Getting to Know the Chesapeake

If Huntington Inn is the freighter model of assisted living (as described in Chapter 4), then the Chesapeake is the cruise ship. We were more than sympathetic to the care supervisor who lamented that neither she, nor, sadly, her mother, could ever afford to live there.

Geographical Place

The Chesapeake is situated between two heavily traveled suburban roads, a half block inward from a major four-lane thoroughfare lined with shopping centers, restaurants, office buildings, and other sundry commercial establishments. Bordering the home on its west side are the public library and a large Christian church complex. The property is esthetically pleasing and the grounds are meticulously maintained, with seasonal plantings of tulips, begonias, or pansies and mature trees shading surrounding paths and parking spaces. A sidewalk encircles the complex, and paths dovetail into open spaces by the library and church and run adjacent to a fenced yard designed for the dementia residents. Lining the sidewalk are a swing, the occasional bench, and age-appropriate exercise stations installed by a partnership between the Chesapeake, a local church, and a hospital.

The suburban community surrounding the Chesapeake is prosperous, white, and educated, much like Dr. Catherine. Residents and families frequently select the Chesapeake because of its reputation, appearance, location, and proximity to family members. Often either relatives or friends live in the area; for some the Chesapeake is the convenient central location to which residents' children, residentially scattered, can travel. In general, residents or their families reflect, or aspire to, the community's social indicators.

Constructed in the 1990s, the Chesapeake is composed of two separate multistoried buildings, one designed for independent living and the other for assisted living, connected by a raised overpass. It is part of a large for-profit chain oriented toward the new assisted living philosophy. The assisted living portion of the Chesapeake accommodates 100 residents, with 40 of these individuals housed in the dementia care unit. Vacancies fill quickly, and the building consistently operates at full capacity.

Social Space

The adjoining church owns the land on which the Chesapeake was built. Part of the rent paid by the corporation provides a resident subsidy program administered through a board composed of church members and a director from the Chesapeake. Residents who have "spent down" their funds request support, and successful applicants have part of their fees paid by the church. No Medicaid residents are accepted, and during our tenure, to save money, several residents moved to military institutions and less expensive homes, into independent living, and "back home" with family. However, the directors try hard to work with families to allow residents to age in place. Dr. Catherine had shrewdly invested her savings and was financially comfortable, facing no risk of displacement.

Like most of its competitors, the Chesapeake is certified for level 3 care, the highest level recognized by the state. Clare feels that the dining room experience is critical to residents' acceptance of the assisted living facility as their home. The Chesapeake therefore does not accept newcomers with medical needs such as feeding tubes that would prevent the shared dining experience. She is also concerned with the effect that health issues— for example, a resident's excessive weight or aggressive behavior—have on the direct care staff. When a resident becomes difficult to handle and requires a two-person assist to get in and out of bed or a chair, that resident is either asked to move or to provide additional, private-duty care.

Clare does not, however, quickly dismiss ornery residents. Mrs. Gold constantly complained and, when in her room, repeatedly rang for the staff to attend to some small chore (pick up a tissue, get her gum, or check her Depends). The staff protested to Clare, who took on the role of direct care provider several times, interacting with Mrs. Gold and responding to her calls. She later explained to the staff that the pettiness of Mrs. Gold's requests was to be tolerated as not all residents are docile and pleasant inhabitants. The care staff do work to accommodate residents who return from the hospital and rehab, and they support in-home hospice. Care aides and directors go out of their way for residents for whom they hold special affection, encouraging them to eat by ordering their favorite foods and enlivening their physical appearance with jewelry and makeup. It was not uncommon to hear that a staff member visited a resident in the hospital, the nursing home, or a new assisted living residence.

Inside the Home

The well-kept state of the facility was noteworthy at the Chesapeake. The front entrance is meant to attract, and the brass-handled, wood-paneled doors swing outward, inviting visitors to enter. A private sitting area extends along the inside of the building, flanked on both sides by walls and windows, separating this quiet space—a sort of "inside porch"—from the reception area. Natural light and strategically placed fixtures in conjunction with rich colors such as wine, turquoise, and hunter green along with spotless rugs, unscathed wooden tables, framed and subtle prints, and recently reupholstered furniture evoke the air of a residential hotel. The directors often introduced some new amenity like an exterior wood-burning stove, Bose speakers mounted outside above the drive-through overhang, and a jukebox in the café.

The lobby was habitually busy, a hub of congregating residents; it even sometimes hinted at chaos, as nearly every resident and employee, and all visitors, passed through this space each day. The receptionist sat at her desk while she answered the telephone, fielded residents' questions, hooked a woman's necklace around her arthritic neck, took orders for the weekly restaurant excursion, discussed weekend plans with the executive director, monitored the television remote control, and reminded forgetful residents about daily schedules. Some residents took to napping in the lobby despite the din, and when other residents and staff complained that snoring women were not in keeping with the Chesapeake's image, all but one chair were removed by the maintenance staff.

Direct care staff members run up and down the grand staircase, just to the left of the reception desk, too busy to take the elevator amid walkers, wheelchairs, and pets. The entrance to the dementia care unit is through an alcove in the rear of the first floor, directly in line with the front door. When a code is pressed into the security keypad, walls separate, facilitating passage. Off the lobby to the right is a café where residents can grab a cookie or a piece of fruit, pour coffee, or get a bowl of cereal; and beyond is the dining room with fresh flowers set on the tables. To the left of the lobby is a television lounge, separated from the reception desk by a wall dominated by a large fish tank, and a hall of suites. On the second floor, four corridors of suites extend from a large and sunny lounge, as do the activities room, small offices and workrooms, the Wellness Center, and the hair salon.

The resident suites include small single-bedroom and two-bedroom units; most are private, but residents have the option of sharing rooms and/or baths. While we were there, residents changed suites because a "nicer" place opened up, because they needed to save money, or because the death of a spouse prompted downsizing to protect future assets.

Throughout the Chesapeake, attractive sitting areas offer residents comfortable public spaces to congregate, extending their small apartments into common living rooms. Residents bring furniture and mementos from home. Dr. Smith brought a work table and tools to craft airplane models; Mrs. Ferraro connected a computer to keep up with friends, surf the Web, and download knitting patterns; and Mr. Peters set up as much acoustical equipment as he could fit to play operas. Most residents have a television, a few with large screens. Residents buy groceries on the weekly food run to the supermarket, and some families deliver snacks and necessities. This enables people to eat in the privacy and comfort of their rooms, where several use coffee pots and microwave ovens. This allows them to indulge in food that the Chesapeake's chef does not cook (though some residents say that they should be reimbursed for meals skipped).

Residents are, however, carefully monitored by the staff to make sure that no one is skipping too many dinners.

Spending Time

On most days, the Chesapeake is lively. Bingo, entertainment from school groups, manicures, exercise classes, Bible lessons, birthday parties, sing-alongs, apple pie socials—an innumerable array of activities are planned to help residents fill their days. Monthly paper calendars are printed and distributed, and some residents keep them close at hand in their purses or walker bags; there is also an electronic daily calendar near the elevator. Family members pass in and out picking up relatives for medical appointments, shopping, and lunch. Several residents go off on their own beyond the grounds. Mrs. Krensky pushed her oxygen tank on her wheelchair when walking to the library; Dr. Smith drove his motorized scooter to the pharmacy; and volunteers chauffeured Mrs. Cooper to her church to count the Sunday collection and Ms. Dobson to a local elementary school to teach reading. Special events are planned throughout the year; the spring dance with nearby uniformed military personnel is a perennial hit, as are the Valentine dinner, the Mother's Day Tea, and the annual Christmas extravaganza, with band, wine bar, and scrumptious finger foods.

Unless tired or unwell, many residents spend large segments of their day walking around the Chesapeake, talking to other residents and the staff. Clare realizes that some residents have never been gregarious and says she doesn't expect them to change now that they have moved into assisted living. Mrs. Drake adopted a pattern of walking outside around the Chesapeake at least seven times a day to keep in shape. She was trying to combat the image visualized in one of her pet phrases, "golden age gone rusty." There are a few whose desire to remain solitary between meals is respected.

Dr. Catherine felt it important to become involved in the Chesapeake. "I like being helpful to people, and there are a lot of people who really need some cheering up." She bundled her own cigarettes in threes for a resident forced to collect and smoke butts off the pavement because the other woman's daughter refused her permission to smoke, and she visited with a blind neighbor who she felt was ignored by her daughter. Almost from the beginning of her move Dr. Catherine contrived an activity whereby residents in the assisted living wing would interact with people in the dementia care unit, keeping company or offering support. She described the lack of social interaction in that unit: "All my friends sit like stones, all in a row." Regarding her proposed activity, "If we ever get this . . . thing off the ground, it will be wonderful."

The Chesapeake, while vocally in favor of her project, had no resources to help with this activity. Dr. Catherine tried to get her neighbors and dining partners on board, but only two steadfastly committed. Dr. Catherine was surprised to find that residents and their families feared dementia. One woman on her corridor expressed interest in participating in visits to the dementia unit until her daughter heard about it. Dr. Catherine related the story: "I had this one lady who was so gung ho about it . . . and her daughter said, 'Oh, no—she can't go near those people. No, no, no—she can't go—we're not going to allow her to go near those people.' It's as if they think it's contagious. I felt terrible. . . . However, I said to them, 'You know, of course that's your decision and choice,' and it's not something we can force on anyone. . . . They must have had a very serious talk with her because . . . she said, 'Oh, no, no—I can't go in there. I can't go in there.' You can't force it."

No One Is Typical

While we were at the Chesapeake, we met residents spanning 60 years in age, in couples and as singles, all with varying backgrounds and reasons for moving there. Several residents had moved into the Chesapeake when it opened, a few came for respite, others tried assisted living and relocated to the independent apartments (several made the transition between independent and assisted living more than once), several relocated, a few entered a nursing home or died, and a few quietly but quickly were channeled into the dementia care unit. The more time we spent at the Chesapeake, the more we appreciated Clare's philosophy that each resident is different, which helps to explain the fact that many of the Chesapeake's rules and policies are malleable.

Staff members varied in ages and backgrounds as well, from young women right out of high school to Gina in her fifties. Some were attending college and were working part time; others focused on full-time work and their families. Several held two jobs. Care aides stopped in on their days off to visit and help when they were in the neighborhood, brought in their children on school holidays, or ran an occasional errand for a resident. The Chesapeake promotes employment advancement from within, and during our tenure we observed a cook, care aides, a housekeeper, and a business assistant promoted to higher positions, and also an upward shifting of positions in marketing, human resources, reception, and care supervision. We also observed as staff members quit and new people began working; however, here at the Chesapeake, employee turnover was not as much an ongoing concern as elsewhere in assisted living facilities.

A Cut Above

The Chesapeake prides itself on its reputation. As symbols of status, the managers wear business casual, and direct care staff members dress in slacks and Chesapeake-monogrammed shirts. Professional grounds crews maintain the landscaping. Directors sustain contact with local aging agencies and associations and are active in regional corporate meetings. The Chesapeake focuses on safety, with technological solutions to monitor potential problems: direct care staff carry beepers and cell phones, residents wear wandering alert bracelets, and residents' telephones signal for help if bumped off the cradle for too long. The staff check on residents every two hours during the night, but a resident can opt out by signing a consent form that is also signed by the resident's family. The corporation mandates that all employees be English-speaking so that they can quickly respond in an emergency.

Appearance was a central and crucial factor in Dr. Catherine's daughter selecting the Chesapeake. In her interview, Susan told us: "Mom's biggest fear in life has always been that she would end up in a nursing home, and so that was the other reason I think that the Chesapeake so appealed to me because it tries so hard to not look like that. And it's not."

Life at the Chesapeake

Even with all of the Chesapeake's activities, residents' lives revolve around meal times. Almost everyone is on time, many congregating beforehand in the nearby lobby, café, or TV lounge. Direct care staff encourage early line-up partly because their job is to cue the forgetful about the upcoming meals, and to walk and wheel those needing help to the dining room. When the staff are in place to take orders and serve, the rope is pulled back, allowing the flood of residents to find their seats.

Residents are assigned seats to minimize disagreements. The shift supervisor places new residents with those she believes to have compatible personalities; if there is dissension or preference, the supervisor makes a change. Residents' photographs posted on a board directly inside the kitchen area help staff members learn faces and names.

Some residents seem tolerant of dementia and physical disability and help each other. Mrs. Krensky was solicitous over her blind tablemate, helping to cut her food, while at another table three women kept Mrs. Martin afloat and out of the dementia care unit by making sure she ate and directing her toward social activities. This is not to say that conflicts did not occur, but the most raucous individuals were placed at tables for two to avoid disturbances and allow the meals to flow smoothly.

Not only did residents come to meals regularly, but also food was a popular topic of conversation. In addition to a resident council, the Chesapeake had a food committee, which held monthly meetings with the assistant director and the chef, offering suggestions and making complaints. Despite this system, the two most vocal members told us that "nothing ever gets done." The chef did solicit recipes from the residents; although he claimed to have made them, no residents recognized them. The chef also attended resident council meetings, but to the annoyance of the most actively engaged residents, some who attend merely sit in silence, preferring to grumble quietly during meals rather than complain publicly at a gathering. Although Dr. Catherine referred to the topics at the council meetings as "mundane," she still participated in "gripe sessions" over menu options, portion sizes, and speed of service.

Companionship

Attachments develop among residents and staff, friendships blossom, and occasionally couples form. Dr. Smith and Mr. Peters became Dr. Catherine's two closest companions; all three were opera aficionados and well-traveled. They conversed in the smoking room and watched operatic videos in Mr. Peters' suite, imbibing alcohol that Dr. Smith purchased and Mr. Peters' family provided. When Dr. Catherine requested a change of seat in the dining room to be with them, she was criticized by Mrs. Mitchell for wanting "to sit with the Ph.D.s" and ridiculed by a staff member for wanting "to sit with the men." Eventually they did share a table in the dining room along with Mrs. Cooper, an amiable woman who had lived one block from the Chesapeake for all of her working life.

Mr. Peters, a recent widower, sent Dr. Catherine flowers, made sexual overtures, invited her to vacation on the beach, and hinted at marriage. Although flattered by his advances, Dr. Catherine was alarmed by Mr. Peters' verbally abusive manner, and she questioned the nature of his attention. Dr. Smith became the closer and more stable friend, sharing her interest in the dementia care unit. He and his wife had entered the Chesapeake together, an arrangement forced on them by their son. Dr. Smith's health was failing, and he had not noticed that his wife was showing signs of dementia. Soon after their move into the Chesapeake, his wife was transferred to the dementia care unit without consulting him and was then moved to a facility specializing in dementia care beyond that provided at the Chesapeake. He and Dr. Catherine voiced essentially the same history; both had been placed in assisted living by their children without their input. Dr. Smith was philosophical about the residents and assisted living:

> Most of the people here . . . have a story, and the story has a sameness about it. They have been placed here by younger relatives who are either unable or uninclined to give them the kind of care that they need and they have been—Are you familiar with the term "warehousing?"—and they've turned over their powers of attorney to their kids and had their homes sold. And they get frequent visits, some more often than others, from their kids. But if you were to sit out here on Sunday on a nice day, and just watch the number of people who go out Sunday morning and come back about 3:00 o'clock in the afternoon—you know, their kids have done their duty. They have given service to what they regard as being necessary duties to their parents, and they're good for another week. [Dr. Smith chuckled.] I think that this business of sticking superannuated people into a cloistered environment is relatively new. People used to look after their elderly people. Every family had a maiden aunt, who looked after

Father or Grandfather or somebody. But it's a whole different climate now.

The Independent Dependent

As described in Chapter 1, resident independence is a touted value of the new assisted living philosophy. Of the six assisted living residences we studied, the management at the Chesapeake is perhaps the most vocal about its commitment to this value. Yet "independence" is framed in ways that people outside assisted living might not recognize. For example, residents' abilities to make decisions are constrained by their own families and the assisted living staff and management.

The Chesapeake, like most assisted living settings, does not provide new residents with an orientation guidebook to help them learn the rules. Dr. Catherine early on felt the pressure of living in an institution. "I think everybody does feel that they're kind of locked up. They're watched for all kinds of things. After the first meal I had here, I went out for a walk and I walked a long time, and they had two people out finding me. And I'm so used to walking and doing those things that I was kind of horrified that I just couldn't go out and walk." She soon learned that she was not permitted to walk to the nearby shopping center or church. "We're really not supposed to do that. . . . When they were out following me, I didn't know I was doing anything wrong. I was just going for a big walk. I thought, oh, my gosh—what is this—they are running after me!" "Oh, I know," she added, "they are all liable and there are all those issues that they have to live with too." Dr. Smith, in a later interview, emphasized this idea. "Most of the residents here are fairly independent. They walk around this place, but they have a—I don't know—they must have some kind of spy network or something that catches people who are trying to cross the road and stuff. They do come down on people who are trying to beat the system." Other residents described similar experiences.

For Dr. Catherine, weekly field trips to local restaurants, organized by the Chesapeake, became one of her few opportunities to exert command over her life similar to the position of power she held in education. On one of these excursions she corralled the maintenance director to argue for installing an air filter in the smoking room, and regularly at lunch outings she ordered wine or cocktails, ostensibly prohibited to her at the Chesapeake because of her alcohol abuse.

Other residents, too, exercised freedom in personal ways. Mr. Peters boasted publicly of his trips to buy liquor and cigars; another confided that she sidestepped the supermarket and "ran into" the adjacent clothing store on a recent grocery run. A resident purchased liquid soap for washing lingerie (detergent is defined as a chemical, needing signed consent to keep in a suite); and Dr. Smith, at first skeptical when his son presented him with a motorized scooter ("What would I ever do with one?"), soon found himself "enchanted" with it: "It has opened up a whole new world for me just to be able to get out of this place. Four walls, you know, can be very oppressive." Initially Dr. Smith imagined that residents might be jealous or resent his "special toy." But, he reported, "It's been just the opposite. I have been very nicely surprised."

Dr. Catherine, too, was happy for her friend ("He gets to go out and do his man thing"), but the gradual loss of independence stalked her. She challenged the Chesapeake's policy that the receptionist distribute only single cigarettes to residents. As noted earlier, residents are not permitted to keep cigarettes in their suites. Rather than handing over her carton, she sometimes kept it: "I'm supposed to, but I told them I'm a little bit too old for that. I don't need to do that, thank you. They haven't forced me to do it." (In reality, staff members comb residents' suites looking for contraband.) Dr. Smith, in a separate interview, commented, "I had to beg from the receptionist two cigarettes at a time." His son ordered a delivery of beer and cigarettes from a local establishment, but they were intercepted at the desk. The smoking policy is intended to provide smokers with options while still protecting the safety of the larger group—one of the restrictions imposed by group living that some assisted living residents find difficult to accept.

Dr. Catherine objected to other policies at the Chesapeake, one being that Tammy, the activities director, had to pay for purchases on the weekly supermarket run. This policy denies residents control over their money and the privacy of their purchases. Another policy restricts over-the-counter medications in the suites. "I bought an extra thing of Tylenol at the grocery store, and Tammy said, 'You have to put that in the nurse's office,' and I said, 'I don't choose to do that.'" Sometimes the nurse would be sent to a resident's room to ask for the over-the-counter drug. She didn't always get it. (Several residents showed us where their caches of over-the-counter drugs were hidden.)

Six months into living at the Chesapeake Dr. Catherine stated, "You see, one of the things I resent about this place—or any place like it—is that it takes away one's independence."

Risk-Taking

Making policy is an ongoing task for the Chesapeake management, especially policies that concern risk. Residents and/or families may be asked to sign negotiated risk agreements that permit the resident to do things that conflict with facility policies. The risk agreement specifies the management's concern and asks the resident and his or her family to accept responsibility for risks associated with the resident's actions. For example, negotiated risk agreements were written for such behavior as "wandering" and refusing to use a monitoring bracelet, refusal of the every-two-hour nightly bed checks, walking to a nearby shopping center, drinking alcohol, and storing cleaning chemicals (i.e., hand laundry detergent) in rooms. As assistant executive director, Clare looks at each individual case and resident before making an agreement, and maintains that there are no hard-and-fast rules: each case is "negotiated." Regarding walking off the grounds, she said: "You know . . . if I have a resident who is not confused and feeling O.K. with it—I let them go. I have a resident who just moved in—he lives . . . kind of right around the corner. That's where his house is—and he and his wife just moved in and every, almost every day he walks over to his old house—and his daughter says that is fine with her. If it's fine with her, it's fine with me. And he did sign—the daughter did sign—a risk form on that."

One son we interviewed was of two minds about allowing his mother to cross the street. On the one hand, she had lived one block from the Chesapeake for close to 50 years and knew the perils of the roadways. On the other hand, she had both depression and dementia and had recently lost her husband. The idea that she might attempt suicide plagued him. He chose not to sign, and his mother was not permitted to walk across the busy street.

Mr. Peters was the first resident to bring a motorized scooter into the Chesapeake. Much to Clare's chagrin, he took it everywhere, from the neighborhood liquor store to the four-lane commercial highway. One time he ran out of charge and sat along the road until he was spotted, by chance, by one of the Chesapeake's marketing staff. Clare noted, "I had a meeting with his family about this and they signed a negotiated risk agreement, saying, 'Our Dad is free to come and go as he pleases . . . We understand he takes his wheelchair—or his motorized vehicle out and that's fine with us.'" When Dr. Smith received his motorized scooter several months later, a facility policy for its use outside the building was firmly in place.

To Barry, the executive director, the Chesapeake is a "managed risk community." Risk taking is acceptable if residents are to retain any independence. He explains. "It's a gray world. . . . A lot of things can happen. . . . [Am I] willing to take those risks to give those residents the independence . . . for them to live out the rest of their life the way they want to?" He is. For Barry, it is the family's and the resident's right to choose the level of risk, as long as that level is within Chesapeake corporate policy. It is "their right of how they choose to live and what environment they want. . . . I mean, anything can happen, and that's what we mean by managed risk. And we're very honest with the families; anything can happen here." Barry went on to give examples, such as tripping over potted plants and knickknacks. "But at least you know we're going to do everything we can to manage that risk." As Clare commented, "There is only so much you can do."

As Dr. Catherine's health improved in the first few weeks she lived at the Chesapeake, she questioned her move and the appropriateness of having to live there. She realized that her daughter wanted her safe after her fall. "But I keep telling her now—I'm fine now and there is no reason for me to be here. And that's what everybody says in the place. They all say— why are you here?" At that time, her dementia was not readily noticeable to other residents; partly because of her intelligence and her sociability, she was able to compensate for her increasing confusion. But over time, that changed.

The Second Transition

From the time Dr. Catherine moved in, the people closest to her knew that she would most likely be relocated eventually to the dementia care unit. Her daughter, Susan, had considered the probable transition when selecting the Chesapeake. Clare, as assistant executive director, has sufficient experience in the field to predict the outcome, and Dr. Catherine herself related her encounter with a psychiatric social worker who told her that she would have severe dementia eventually. For Clare, this transitional process was exceptionally long and complex because Dr. Catherine is such a "unique case." Her transition was "hard" because she was often "so lucid" and "sometimes she's so good."

Clare finds families challenging and difficult to convince when the staff at the Chesapeake decides it is time for their relatives' move into the dementia care unit. Despite documented assessments and agreement on entry, Susan, too, questioned the timing when Clare suggested that the move was imminent. Residing in assisted living allows the family hope for stability; movement into the dementia care unit forces them to recognize and accept their relative's decline. Once in dementia care, residents rarely leave.

As assisted living coordinator, Richard is quick to pick up on the frequency of denial by both families and residents. Reasons for transitioning need to be documented and warranted by the staff "because you have to justify [the move] to the family, because the family doesn't want to see Mom and Dad decline." As for residents, "it's so hard when you're dealing with the human mind . . . they don't want to see themselves decline. Some of them understand and get frustrated by the fact that they are declining. A lot of them sink into a depression because of that."

Dr. Catherine's second transition, the one into dementia care, slowly progressed over three years. She demonstrated confusion in lighting cigarettes, using eating utensils, and finding her place in the dining room. She needed direction to her suite, a short walk from the television lounge, and she lit a match next to an oxygen tank, to the horror of its owner, Mrs. Krensky. Susan hired dog walkers, and when their twice-daily visits proved inadequate, direct care aides walked Muffin. Clare planned early on for both Muffin's and Dr. Catherine's transition together into the dementia care unit, but the dog required too much of the staff's time, and, to Dr. Catherine's great sadness, Muffin was adopted by her walkers. As time went on, Dr. Catherine disrobed in public, had frequent toileting accidents, demonstrated an inability to communicate with other residents, displayed problems with eating, and talked to what she believed was another person in the mirror. She was repeatedly evaluated by the staff, and reports were made regularly to Susan.

Dr. Catherine's physical condition also gradually changed. She put on weight, her breathing was sometimes labored, and her walking slowed when she began to drag her feet. There was also a decline in her balance, ability to walk straight, and lower body strength. She rested frequently and intermittently while walking about the Chesapeake, and negotiating stairs became increasingly problematic.

Dr. Catherine had been a visible resident since her move-in, spending at least as much time outside her suite as in it. Over time, Mrs. Krensky, Mrs. Mitchell, and Mrs. Randall, all active residents at the Chesapeake, began to comment on her decline. Shouldn't she be "back there," Mrs. Krensky wondered, referring to the dementia care unit? When Dr. Catherine left for a visit to her daughter's home, Mrs. Mitchell assumed she had moved into the dementia unit; she wondered what life was like "back there" but never initiated a visit to see it for herself. Other residents were more kind, helping her along in getting wherever she needed to go. Mr. Peters had long since left the Chesapeake for another assisted living facility, and Dr. Smith, perhaps because of depression or embarrassment, or because Dr. Catherine's decline resembled his wife's, ignored her. Dr. Catherine had either forgotten or disregarded the service program that previously excited her and stopped visiting friends in the dementia care unit. When her neighbor moved there, Dr. Catherine explained the transition as one in which Mrs. Wood "graciously" accommodated her daughter's wishes. Hearing this comment caused us to wonder if Dr. Catherine anticipated her own move.

The one problematic issue that Susan had with the Chesapeake was the staff's inability to control her mother's drinking, especially because her dementia was alcohol-related. The staff told Susan the drinking could be discouraged but not curtailed, as it occurred in other residents' rooms. Richard, the assisted living coordinator, agreed to be the "enforcer" because drinking caused a month-long rift with her mother whenever Susan brought up the topic. Susan also appreciated Richard's offer to make a policy specifically addressing Dr. Catherine's problems. (In an interview, Richard told us that his goal is to make families' lives easier.)

Over the years we were in contact with the Chesapeake, Clare worked with Susan to prepare for her mother's transition, and called their relationship "close." Susan finally agreed to the move if a suite opened in the dementia care unit that was identical to the one her mother lived in outside its walls; this, she felt, would make for a seamless adjustment. When one became available, Clare felt the time was right, and Susan and her brother agreed. Dr. Catherine "loved" her new room and "was fine with moving." After the first week, she no longer expressed any interest to leave the unit.

I visited with Dr. Catherine after her move. She had lost weight and her breathing was regular. I am sure she remembered me, not as the researcher who interviewed her but as a friendly face somewhere from the past. She asked about my family and told me stories about the people sitting around us, many of whom I knew; I recalled Dr. Smith saying that everyone has a story. Later, as we walked down a hallway toward her room—she was eager to show it off—I found her slow and unsteady and wondered about her using a walker. I felt she could possibly fall, as she clutched my arm tightly. I asked a care staff member how far down the hall did Dr. Catherine live. "Dr. Catherine?" In surprise, she asked, "Dr. Who?" Dr. Catherine's title did not follow her into the dementia care unit, nor was she leading me in the right direction. Catherine lived on the other side of the wing.

Final Thoughts

Values

Independence is a core tenet in assisted living philosophy. The popular definition of independence as freedom of choice, however, cannot always be realized in assisted living. Residents who have cognitive impairments and physical disabilities must rely on others, including their families and the assisted living staff, for guidance and direct care. Dr. Catherine was clear in telling us that assisted living stripped her of that valued trait, with "independence" meaning little more than menu choice and degree of participation in social activities, yet she did bring her dog to the Chesapeake and made decisions about what she did and with whom on a daily basis—as long as she did not leave the property unescorted and conformed to the implied rules in the assisted living setting. Safety and independence are trade-offs viewed differently by residents, family members, and administrators.

In our interviews with families and staff, the topic of safety frequently surfaced. Certainly safety is important, but the degree of protection promoted by the family and/or staff can be at odds with the residents' preferences. Susan described safety as a prime concern in selecting the Chesapeake. Even Dr. Catherine herself realized that problems of risk exist, yet her very sense of self was as a capable and independent woman. Accepting the limitations imposed by assisted living staff, management, and her daughter presented an ongoing adjustment for her.

Lifestyle Change

By its very nature, assisted living is an institutionalized residential setting, in some ways antithetical to the ways of life residents held before they entered. After living a private and sometimes solitary life before assisted living, residents at the Chesapeake interact on a regular basis in close quarters with more than one hundred other people. They must adapt to loss of privacy, for people enter their rooms unannounced, and the staff either open doors and knock (in that order) or use a key to gain entrance at will. Mrs. Podesta, a woman with whom we spoke often, lamented one afternoon that her reputation was "ruined." Tammy, the activities director, had observed her drinking a glass of wine, assumed she was inebriated, related the incident to the entire second-floor staff, and sent a letter to her son. She eventually signed her own risk agreement to drink two ounces of alcohol per night to help her sleep. The accommodation to assisted living requires adjustment to a new physical space, a changing lifestyle, and an aging body, all at the same time.

At the Chesapeake, assisted living is a cross between a private home, a residential hotel, and a medical clinic. Meals are served in an elegant dining room, and residents collect for small talk in the lobby. However, as Mrs. Wood commented one morning, "If this is my home, why can't I come to breakfast in my bathrobe?" Learning what signifies home or hotel, another lifestyle change, is sometimes confusing and rarely rational.

Another example of the public nature of private behavior involves Mrs. Drake. One afternoon when she ran into the café wearing a pink housecoat to retrieve a sweater she realized she had left behind, the care staff questioned her cognition based on her decision to appear in public in her nightgown!

Although not a nursing facility, an assisted living residence by necessity involves medical care. The emphasis on wellness belies its true nature, that of caring for residents' health needs and dispensing of medications on a regular basis privately in rooms and publicly in lounges and the dining room. Relying on a medical technician to receive pills in view of other residents and staff, a true lifestyle change, might further erode some residents' sense of independence by making a private act a public occurrence.

Communication in assisted living is also compromised. Residents of the Chesapeake bemoan not being kept informed on the whereabouts and health status of their friends and neighbors. They complain that no one takes heed of what they say at council and committee meetings and feel these gatherings are a sham. Residents also deliberately hide signs of decline to maintain an identity as a fit and functioning person and avoid paying higher fees for increased levels of care.

Resident Transitioning

We found the residential population at the Chesapeake to be diverse and somewhat transient. We interviewed residents ranging in age from 49 to 104. These people came from varying occupations, educational levels, and geographic backgrounds. Although in assisted living facilities many individuals decline and go to the hospital or skilled nursing, we also noted that some residents remained stable. Several do remain for years in one long-term care setting. Others move back home (mostly with relatives), into independent living, to another assisted living or group home, or to another institution offering a different type of care, such as a dementia care facility. After three years, the youngest woman residing at the Chesapeake, Ms. Dobson, a teacher who had been in a car accident, defied all odds and moved, with her service dog, into a townhome accessible to her motorized chair and near a supermarket.

Residents who leave do so mostly on their own volition; some, however, are asked to leave because they have not paid their bills, have spent down their funds, have increased medical needs, exhibit aggression or in-tolerable behavior, or refuse movement into the dementia care unit. Some are asked to leave because they refuse to accept services. Clare said she has had many conversations with residents about their negative attitudes toward the staff and has tried to explain that "they are here to help you." If the situation becomes uncontrollable, she has no problem discharging residents.

Families are encouraged to plan for the future. Dr. Catherine's daughter Susan, despite all her preparations for her mother's care, found that finalizing decisions was difficult. Even after hiring an elder care consultant, visiting assisted living homes, and talking with friends, she felt at odds with the process. She concluded that there is no good, reliable way of getting a family member situated. Speaking about her mother's move into assisted living, Susan said: "When I was younger I couldn't understand why it seems to happen this way. When you hear of people's stories, so often . . . there's some calamity that occurs, and then there is a crisis and you have to do everything in a crisis. And that seems so stupid, when it could be something that you could plan for, and you could plan for it together, and everyone could have a say, you know, in the decision making. My understanding now is that, I now understand why it never works that way, or seldom works that way, because I can understand the older family member wants to maintain themselves in their own home. And until there is proof positive that they can't, which usually comes in the form of a calamity, then you're at odds. And so I don't see that there is usually a positive planful way to do this."

The Goal of the Chesapeake

An assisted living residence is often defined by what it isn't—a nursing home. Clare remarked in one interview that nursing homes have a nega-tive reputation, and we heard this repeatedly from families, residents, and staff. Assisted living, she pointed out, "has a reputation of being nicer, homier, more comfortable than nursing homes," and she speaks of it as a good option for individuals seeking long-term care.

Who does well at the Chesapeake? According to Clare, those who do are the "social butterflies like the Ms. Mitchells and the Ms. Woods, and the, you know, people that like—even someone like Glenda Martin, who's so pleasantly confused, but loves to be around people, loves interaction. Those types of people, I think do really well. Although you have your apartment, it's still not a private place. They're eating with all these people. . . . you have care aides in and out of your room checking on you, and I mean, there's a lot of commotion. There's a lot going on. So I think the people that thrive on having company and so forth do well here."

Despite the apparent emphasis placed on family-administration oversight and communication, Clare and Barry, directors at the Chesapeake, both feel that the residents are their main clients, and they echo corporate philosophy to meet residents' needs. "My goal," maintains Clare, "is to make sure that the residents are happy." Although families need to be satisfied, "number one, first and foremost, are residents."

SEVEN

Mr. Sidney at Laurel Ridge

I sat in my car in the small parking lot facing the entrance to Laurel Ridge. I found the building attractive in the late morning sun, and although there is minimal landscaping—six red geraniums in the summer or six purple pansies in the fall, interspersed with a few hardy and drought-resistant greens—the tall lush trees overlooking the grounds from the adjoining property give a parklike feel to the home. A large mobility transport van backed up and pulled away, probably taking someone to dialysis or a doctor's appointment, and the ice cream delivery truck drove out a little too fast for my comfort. Mr. Howard's sister pulled up alongside me, smiled and nodded, and grabbed his laundry from the trunk. (Mr. Howard, in his early fifties, has a brain tumor, and one of his eight siblings in their staunch Catholic family takes a turn visiting each day, shuttling him to the Basilica for walks and minding his care.) I reminded myself that I needed to select a resident on which to focus, to write about. Each resident has a compelling story. I sat there asking myself: whom should I pick? I had been ruminating on this question for weeks.

After gathering my notebook and tape recorder from the front seat, I spotted Mr. Sidney in his wheelchair, sitting off to the side of the front door, head back, enjoying the sun. "God's signature" is how he described the clouds to me one afternoon. He was dressed to "go out," never leaving his room without a jacket, sports cap, and waist pack, no matter the weather. He is always polite, pleasant, and pensive, and I thought of him often speaking positively of life from his perch of ninety-seven years. From Mr. Sidney I have learned to appreciate a calm approach to life and death, and I am grateful for his willingness to share in the research. I decided that Mr. Sidney's life would make for a fine story.

We first interviewed Mr. Sidney in the spring of 2005, four and a half months after he moved to Laurel Ridge. We had already met several times, and he could always be found at exercise class at ten in the morning or at the discussion or word game afterward. Exercise is what is "very good" about Laurel Ridge, he said; it tests not only the body but also the mind. "Some do it," he said, "to live longer." He did it "to feel better; it keeps me alive."

Mr. Sidney attended all activities with Mrs. Perkins, a resident he met within days of his arrival. They ate together, kept company, and "watch[ed] out for each other." Staff at Laurel Ridge referred to them as a "couple"; an observant nurse told us, "they talk." Drawn together as two of the few cognitively astute residents, they both had lost spouses, were childless, and had few close living relatives. Mrs. Perkins had one niece who orchestrated her care. Della, the great-niece of Mr. Sidney's second wife, handled his finances, purchased groceries and medical supplies, and brought him to her home for holidays and special events. Mr. Sidney called Della his "guardian angel" and acknowledged the good care she provided.

In this chapter we discuss an expanded notion of what it means to be family and the part "fictive kin" play in resident oversight. We examine what life is like in a locked setting, where residents with severe dementia freely roam throughout the home; the effect a financially stressed and census-challenged assisted living facility has on its population; how ethnicity is perceived; and the notion of friendship in the lives of residents at Laurel Ridge.

Introducing Mr. Sidney

Mr. Sidney exuded a commanding presence. A tall man, even in his wheelchair, he appeared fit. He recognized that his memory was failing and his eyes were bad.

"This old mind is kind of tight," he said, and though he was not "jumping up and down," Mr. Sidney found that life was "not too bad." On the table in his room he kept a game board and challenged himself, moving the marbles according to varying strategies, which he said helped keep his mind intact. Although he felt that his body was weakening, he had what his favorite nurse called "a young man mind."

One of three sons in a Navy family, Mr. Sidney moved among several states while growing up, his family finally settling in Washington, DC. College educated and job searching right after the stock market crash of 1929, he eventually joined the military, completing officer's training during World War II. He spoke eloquently yet sorrowfully of the devastation he witnessed on the beaches and bombed sites of Japan. In spite of the war, Mr. Sidney enjoyed living abroad, especially in Australia, but was prompted by his family after the death of his father to return to the States. He took a position with a transportation division of the U.S. Postal Service, which he liked to say was affiliated historically with the Pony Express, and remained there until age 59. For the next six years he worked in retail sales and at the time we interviewed him had been retired for more than 30 years.

Moving to Assisted Living

His great-niece Della and his physician both felt that Mr. Sidney was reaching a point where it was becoming untenable for him to continue living alone for several reasons. He had already given up driving because he found himself going through red lights and had decided to stop "before the cops caught me." He was eating poorly, even by his own admission. His doctor suggested Laurel Ridge as a potential home; Della and her mother knew of it, and they arranged for his move-in. Mr. Sidney eventually and reluctantly agreed. He expected to walk through its doors, but instead, just before leaving the hospital after a routine admission, he fell and hit his head on the edge of a table, giving him a severe blow to his skull. He told us that he was "totally independent" but came to Laurel Ridge "as an invalid from just being a healthy person. I came over here as a cripple." He realized that he would have moved irrespective of the fall, but it grated on him that he was now an invalid: "If I hadn't fell there, I would probably still be in here, but I wouldn't be an invalid."

Most of the time Mr. Sidney found Laurel Ridge to be a "good place" where he was well cared for. The staff, he thought, was "just like family," but as with family, he had issues. The staff was "worked to death," and so he often did not get the help he needed, especially because he looked self-sufficient and rarely voiced concern. He called the place "cheap": "If you're not paying for the best, you can't live by the best," he told us. "This is not a Wisconsin Avenue joint—not by a long shot," referring to a street in Washington, DC, long known for its high-rent status. Mr. Sidney often talked about the frailty of the residents and their apparent low level of physical acuity: "Fifty percent of the people easily are asleep all the time—they sleep in exercise class!" He appreciated having "nursing care" on site 24/7 and having his medications administered but felt that "the medicines . . . should be the best department in here . . . but it's not. It's the worst." (The best department, he asserted, was housekeeping.)

Mr. Sidney was comfortable at Laurel Ridge but wished it would hire fewer foreign staff members. "The help here are all foreigners. Just about all of them . . . and you can't understand them, and they don't stay, and some aren't worth a damn, and you can't get along with them. They should never have a foreigner handling the medicine, and they will do that." This matter of ethnicity and staff surfaced in talk with other residents, family members, and administrators. One resident moved to Laurel Ridge because her previous assisted living home had an "African"-only staff, only to find immigrants here. Another resident, Ms. Clinton, worked with a care aide to lessen the aide's fear of electricity, after finding out that she was too scared to plug in and recharge Ms. Clinton's motorized chair. About this, Ms. Clinton laughed, "Who's assisting who in assisted living!" Barbara, Mrs. Perkins's niece, told us: "Well, some of [the staff members] is hard to understand. They have that thick accent, you know—most of them are from another country. And I think sometimes, you know—there are certain cultures don't give a lot of empathy to older patients . . . they figure—you're old—you're just old. . . . Some cultures think that when you get old—you know, this is it. You don't need all that care. . . . They don't have the warm bedside manner. . . . But I find . . . if you complain too much on them, they sort of like stand off from you."

Dolores, the executive director at Laurel Ridge, has worked in long-term care for more than 30 years, with experience in both nursing homes and assisted living facilities. Trained in nursing, she prefers the business and administrative side of running a home, and has worked in the for-profit and nonprofit sectors, including as executive director for the corporation that owns the Chesapeake (the assisted living residence discussed in chapter 6). Laurel Ridge "is the first all-black home I've ever had." As an African American herself, she admits to having a difficult time with the cultural differences of her staff, especially regarding eye contact, language, and perceptions of trust. Staff members look down or away when addressed, and they often speak in harsh tones. "They don't mean any harm; they're good people," she says, but family members and residents get upset and think the staff untrustworthy. Laundry is also problematic; staff members don't know what is and is not washable, what should be sent to the dry cleaner, and what should be hand laundered. "You end up doing a lot of . . . in-services and training, and then they'll catch on with what we're doing"—or, as we found out, are instructed by residents on what to do.

Finding Companionship and Settling In

Soon after he moved in—"day 10," Della calculated—Mr. Sidney "hit it off" with Mrs. Perkins. Although the two were considered a couple by the staff, he maintained, "We're just friends." Together they attended activities (although one would go without the other), ate at the same dining table, and monitored each other's health. "She looks out for me and I look out for her." Della called their relationship a "blessing," and Barbara, too, was pleased, though she thought Mr. Sidney was a womanizer, at least in his younger days, and worried about his being a university graduate and athlete. "I think Mr. Sidney picked my aunt . . . because she carries herself . . . and she does have a pretty good mind. . . . I don't know how they clicked; they just started clicking."

Both Mrs. Perkins and Mr. Sidney relied on each other and valued their companionship. The staff knew how much he missed her when she was hospitalized, and when the nurse told him on the day of her return to Laurel Ridge that she was back, he quickly left the library to "give her a ring." In one interview, Mrs. Perkins commented, "I get lonesome." She went on to describe how Mr. Sidney came over to sleep, he in his wheelchair and she in her recliner, keeping each other company. Sometimes she inquired if we had seen her friend that day, as she worried when he missed exercise class or a meal.

Mr. Sidney also talked highly of another dining table companion, Mrs. Waters, who shared his interest in nutritious food. They both took the Laurel Ridge dining staff to task for not keeping water glasses filled or serving salads. Mrs. Waters was quite vocal, reminding the home of its responsibilities to older folk, and shared Mr. Sidney's strong support of exercise. She walked outside around the perimeter of Laurel Ridge several times daily unless the sidewalks were slippery after winter ice storms. Although Mr. Sidney was not gregarious, he did participate in resident council meetings, occasionally played checkers with three of the men, and joined Mrs. Perkins for bingo.

Mr. Sidney seemed ambivalent about his move into an assisted living residence, and specifically to Laurel Ridge. On the one hand, he was aware of his increasing decline and his need for assistance. On the other hand, his preference, like most residents, was to be younger and back in his own home. There were days when he was comfortable, and others when he was "not happy." One afternoon in June eight months after moving in, Laurel Ridge was "beginning to feel like a jail" and he was "terribly bored"; he commented that he needed to "get my life together" and "back on track." A month later he was sorry he had sold his home, felt that he was "quickly talked into this"—referring to selling his house to Della's niece and leaving his old neighborhood. By August, he was more content. He told the interviewer that he now thought of moving only when he got "mad." "I don't think I want to go anywhere else. I'm satisfied here."

Rebecca, the move-in coordinator at Laurel Ridge, says that the hardest thing about transitioning for residents is "losing their home. . . . going from a two-story house to a room." Dolores notes that the settling-in period can last from two months to a year before a person is comfortable in assisted living and feels "this is the place I want to be." However, she is not under any illusions. "There's no place like home. No matter what you do, there's no place like home." There is a conceptual difference between what constitutes the image of "home" and the assisted living room or suite. One afternoon a resident with dementia walked up to the front desk and inquired as to the location of her room. Pleasantly, the receptionist directed her "home." The woman replied that she would love to go home, but since her house had been sold, she would have to be satisfied with her current room.

Doing ethnography at Laurel Ridge was complicated by three factors. First, this two-story building was constructed almost 20 years ago for an independent and mobile population of residents. The corridors are long and form a square around an outside courtyard, and at several points other corridors fan out from this pattern. One small, slow elevator services all of the residents and staff. This design works to keep residents in their rooms. For a frail population, it is a long trip to the front of the building, and there is minimal staff to chauffeur residents to and fro. Consequently, it was difficult to casually meet and converse with residents, which is necessary to establish rapport. Our strategy instead was to knock on residents' doors, resulting often in interrupting naps or television soap operas.

Second, a lounge on the second floor and the library on the first were commandeered by the medical staff to house the medication carts and dispense medicines. The only other public spaces open to residents are the activities room (where, when events are not scheduled, the television is blaring), the downstairs television lounge, and an outside patio used during nice weather. Few residents sought "permission" to exit the front door to sit outside or walk along the parking lot. This, too, made it difficult for us to meet residents outside of planned activities.

Third, the dining room has its own staff. At the Chesapeake, we assisted the direct care aides serving meals and helping residents, and were able to use this interaction to consolidate relationships [see Chapter 6]. At Laurel Ridge, direct care staff were assigned different corridors and residents every six weeks; they spent more time in residents' rooms and less time in the halls because staff census was low and they had more work; and when they could take a break, the aides congregated in or "escaped" to a small staff lounge next to the director of nurses' office. Housekeepers took lunch privately in vacant rooms or in the laundry area. Joseph, the director of nursing, said one afternoon that lunch is often "in a cup," meaning that no one has time to sit and eat, only a moment to grab a drink and take it with her. As a result, our interaction with staff members was limited.

We did, however, take part in activities, painting nails and assisting with crafts and bingo; we attended resident council meetings; and we spent time chatting, outside and in. We visited with residents regularly, learning early on who did and who did not watch the "soaps," and about other daily routines. We also learned early on how important the meal hours were to residents, and we had to juggle our research time accordingly, remembering not the hour set for the meal but the informal time of line-up that happened well in advance of the posted mealtime. We bought items for one woman who found it difficult to leave Laurel Ridge, things like a thimble and stamps. (Trips to the bank and the post office seem to be problematic for assisted living homes, making it difficult for residents to obtain cash and postal supplies.) We helped this same resident get a feel of using a laptop, and brought tools and hung up Mrs. Perkins's photographs. One of our university interns photographed an artist's entire collection of two hundred paintings to categorize for submission to a museum database.

Fieldwork has its playful side. Until he became ill, I regularly met with one man to play checkers. Now 85, he had been playing since he was eight years old, and he and fellow employees played at lunch time during the greater part of their working years. I hadn't played since the age of nine, and he took me from being a neophyte to a winner. Despite his losing to me, I don't know who was more pleased at my winning, him or me. Ironically, on that day, Mrs. Perkins had asked me how I fared. When I told her of my success, she loudly exclaimed, "Go girl!"

Mr. Sidney was almost always ready to talk with us, except in those rare instances when he felt bad. We discussed his health, our families, and his life. We reminisced about his wife, his military exploits, and his work. He often left us with some new insight on the positive side of aging and said how "very lucky" life's treated him.

Getting to Know Laurel Ridge

Although not a "Wisconsin Avenue joint," Laurel Ridge serves a population for which, according to its executive director, the region does not provide: a contingent of middle-class African American residents who have lived in Washington, DC, for most of their working lives.

Geographical Place

Laurel Ridge, part of a small for-profit chain, is situated on a busy four-lane street, divided by a median, on a popular bus route. To the north is a train station and shopping center housing both a Starbucks and a Latin food market. Further north, the street runs adjacent to a major fashion mall and eventually works its way into the outskirts of a university campus. Traveling south, bus riders can step out into a small commercial sector that houses African food marts and ethnic restaurants, or continue on to the adjoining city. Large, private tree-filled lots surround the rest of Laurel Ridge.

The building consists of two stories constructed into a hillside. This makes the inner back core of the first floor unusable for resident living; offices, laundry rooms, and a private dining room are located in this windowless space. The parking lot faces the long front of the building; only a narrow side of the home abuts traffic. Residents sitting out front see neighboring greenery and sky just beyond the short stretch of the parking lot. Because trees and a grassy slope make it difficult for potential consumers to see Laurel Ridge from the main road, the large sign put up by the owners advertising available rentals is the main indicator that an assisted living residence sits on the hill.

Cost, location, and a nurse on duty 24/7 are three factors that may be considered by prospective residents and their families in looking for an assisted living residence. Most of Laurel Ridge's formerly urban residents needed to move out of the city to be near their children's or nieces' suburban homes. The staff at Laurel Ridge markets to community groups and churches, and they have developed a strong network with a nearby hospital, an adult day care center, social workers, ministry outreach, and other assisted living and group homes. Laurel Ridge can accommodate 112 residents; the average number of residents is near 85, but the management would prefer 95.

Social Space

Della found that her uncle's move into assisted living was "good and necessary." Acknowledging Mr. Sidney's recent decline, she appreciated that Laurel Ridge was "hospitable" and "very caring," and, importantly, could provide the care he would need before a possible transition into a nursing home. Della's greatest concern was whether she would have to move him, "which I don't want to do." Like Dr. Smith at the Chesapeake, she referred to nursing homes as "warehouses."

Laurel Ridge is licensed for level 3 care. Residents pay an additional fee for greater assistance. While the home does not accept Medicaid, it does have two internal subsidy programs to help residents age in place. One program gives financially strapped clients reduced rent when moving in, the philosophy being that some income generated for vacant rooms is better than none. There is also a "spend-down" program where residents who have lived at least two years at Laurel Ridge and find themselves out of funds may be charged less. This helps to keep the building's occupancy rate up.

One of Joseph's jobs as director of nursing is to complete assessments on new and continuing residents. Over the years he has found Laurel Ridge taking in and keeping "sicker" residents. "You see people with multiple stroke . . . uncontrollable diabetes . . . respiratory conditions," things "you're not equipped to deal with." These residents, he feels, should be in a nursing home, but they prefer assisted living because it is "as close to home as you can get." Despite this trend in health needs, the number of staff members has not increased to meet demand.

Another characteristic of the social environment of Laurel Ridge is that instead of segregating residents with severe dementia into a special unit, as we saw at Huntington Inn, Middlebury Manor, and the Chesapeake, Laurel Ridge's policy is to lock all of its exits, essentially creating one large, all-inclusive dementia care unit. Family members, visitors, tradespeople, and residents are buzzed in and out, all at the discretion of the receptionist. Residents complained at council meetings and with each other about residents' wandering into their rooms day and night, often staying for long periods of time, taking money and items of clothing, banging on doors, and removing residents' name signs. One administrator described the Laurel Ridge approach as a "rights" issue that supports the freedom of people with dementia to act as they see fit; some staff members felt that working with so diverse a population was stressful and hoped for increased staffing.

Inside the Home

The front door to Laurel Ridge is not disabled-accessible, so after being "buzzed" in, we sometimes were called on to help a resident in a wheelchair or with a walker to exit through the doorway. We also learned which residents needed to be kept from leaving the building. Occasionally it was problematic negotiating both at the same time.

The lobby is large. The receptionist's desk is positioned to allow the receptionist to see the glass front door. Bird cages donated by a postal worker fill one section near the windows. The lobby area originally held chairs, but the staff found that these too often attracted residents with behavioral problems, so they removed the seating. To the right of the lobby as one enters the building is an administrative office, and to the left is the dining room. Straight ahead is a T intersection leading in one direction to a hair salon, copier room, two more administrative offices, and residents' suites, and to the left, a staircase, the "library" (a room with wallpaper depicting book shelves and used for medicine distribution), and more living areas. The building surrounds an outside patio; corridors go off in several directions. On the second level, the activities room is the focal point of resident contact. The nursing station and nursing director's office, the staff and "medication" lounges, and a specialized dining room used to feed and care for frail residents complete the public areas. An additional patio, surrounded on three sides by a high fence, is located outside the rear of the building. It is open to residents only for special events, like the Fourth of July barbecue.

Most residents live in small rooms with private baths. Larger rooms are marketed for two people, defined as either a couple or roommates. In one shared room, Mrs. Jones and her roommate lined up their single beds in front of two individual televisions. Mrs. Jones had no problem sharing the bathroom, she told me, unless it was occupied for too long a time. Mrs. Perkins, on the other hand, "went through" 10 roommates, until the executive director finally gave her a single; the spend-down program helped her family pick up part of the extra cost. Mrs. Perkins had the reputation of being a somewhat difficult resident, called "feisty" by her niece. In her defense, we learned that she had had no previous contact with anyone with severe dementia; she was also placed with women who had behavioral problems, some severe. One roommate frequently took her things; another hit her.

> Mrs. Perkins said her roommate swung her arm at her, knocking her glasses off. She didn't think she was hurt because Mrs. McDonald is so weak and small, but she is still having her eyes checked. . . . Even though Mrs. McDonald didn't do a lot of damage, it has been upsetting and frightening for Mrs. Perkins. She was afraid to go to sleep at night. Joseph, the director of nursing, refused to accept the story. . . . "She didn't hit you," he told her. This really angered Mrs. Perkins. She insists that she was hit. The staff removed Mrs. McDonald from Mrs. Perkins' room on Monday. Both Mr. Sidney and Mrs. Perkins were relieved when she was finally able to have her own suite.

Residents repeatedly described how much they liked the appearance of Laurel Ridge. Dolores, the executive director, believed that the building needs a face lift, but the corporate ownership refused to issue funds for this purpose. The director of maintenance performed small renovations when time permitted—he repainted the guest bathroom during our research—but more often he was kept busy fixing leaking air conditioning units, assembling lawn furniture, replacing light bulbs, and doing everything that a building supervisor accomplishes in an apartment house. When we started the research, the dining room was covered with a dark-colored, stained carpet, and the chairs had wheels. Dolores told us that the carpet needed to be "thrown out, pulled up, burned." Soon after our research was completed, she finally convinced the corporate office to make some changes. A light-colored wood floor was installed, and gliders replaced chair wheels. Linen tablecloths and napkins, vases of flowers, and stemmed glass water goblets remained.

Dolores also thought the corporate office should allot more money toward activities. When we first arrived, there was a full-time, college-trained director of activities working toward professional certification. When the resident census abruptly fell, this position was cut, and several part-time employees periodically took over. Dolores felt that assisted living homes need "pied pipers" to get residents moving and involved. Despite the limited budget, residents enjoyed bingo and Pokeeno, nail polishing, game playing, group television watching, exercise class, and occasional field trips to local stores, the pharmacy, and restaurants. Special events included a yearly trip to a raceway, a Christmas party, monthly birthday celebrations, and a fashion show in May with residents as "stars" modeling clothes from a local shop. Some religious groups hosted dinners for residents at their church halls, and several churches provided services at Laurel Ridge on Saturdays and Sundays with good music and an excellent turnout.

The Average Resident

"Nobody is average," Joseph said in an interview, although when pressured he outlined characteristics of an "ideal type" resident of Laurel Ridge. "I can give you this. Someone who has been at home for a long time and they have been taken care of by the family. . . . The family sees that they cannot meet his needs. . . . He's refusing care. . . . [They bring] him to assisted living. And sometimes the family may be overwhelmed. . . . And they find out it's too much." At Laurel Ridge, residents range in age from people in their early 50s with mental health problems to women over the age of 100 whose major health issue is physical frailty. Many residents have involved families, but others do not. There are also residents who have no family locally or have fictive kin who might be stretched too thin with other demands to provide ongoing assistance. The facility is also home to respite placements and to people who take longer than average in rehabilitation, because developing strength and engaging in physical therapy is less expensive in assisted living than in a skilled nursing setting.

A Cut Below

Competition between assisted living homes is keen. Dolores noted: "What's going for us is that we have the cheapest rates around. I find that consumers are smarter than what they used to be—way smarter." She attributed this to a computer-savvy generation. "There is so much information out there—and you can pull up anything you want. . . . The consumers are very intelligent."

When consumers "pull up" Laurel Ridge on the Internet and then visit in person, they find an assisted living home that has a nurse on duty 24 hours a day, administrators who are willing to work with the financial resources of residents and family members, many services provided in the base monthly price, a convenient location, a partnership with a local hospital and geriatric medical practice, and a staff that is stable, even if few in number and overworked.

Life at Laurel Ridge

In various conversations, Mr. Sidney called his co-inhabitants at Laurel Ridge "residents," "inmates," "tenants," and "patients." This categorization by someone living on the inside fits well with the types of residents we observed and interviewed, and reflects on their lifestyles. Many residents were frail, with multiple health problems, and a good part of their day was spent lining up or sitting and waiting for a nurse to dispense pills. In fact, during the early part of our study there, residents complained that the lines to receive medicine were so long and so slow, and chairs so few, that they often trekked back to their suites to wait for a less-congested time, sometimes making this trip to the medication cart three and four times. Many other residents (and family members) used the word "patient" to describe those living at Laurel Ridge, because they felt that if they were not sick, they would not be living here.

As for "inmates," Mr. Sidney himself told us that Laurel Ridge was "beginning to feel like a jail," though when he used the term "inmates," he followed it with a grin. Residents who were prohibited from leaving, either because they wandered or because the staff feared that they would board the public bus at a nearby stop, undoubtedly did feel constrained. Mr. Caruthers (whom we recognized as having once lived at Huntington Inn) had been known to call a taxi and travel to parts unknown. In fact, he spent a good portion of one Sunday afternoon yelling in the lobby that he wanted to be let out of Laurel Ridge and on his own for the day; finally, the promise of a monetary "bribe" calmed him down. Prison, in this case, is a good analogy for institutional living, with the staff serving as wardens.

The terms "resident" and "tenant" imply independence. "Resident" connotes living at a place without a sense of ownership. Here at Laurel Ridge, some individuals happily went about their day, feeling safe, secure, and contented. "Tenant" speaks to a familiar category of real estate; all residents either rented or held real estate before moving into assisted living. The term implies a monetary exchange with some control and did fit some individuals living at Laurel Ridge. Ms. Clinton paid her own bills and "rented" two rooms, one in which to store her substantial collection of art. Ms. Hart completely remodeled her suite, painting and recarpeting, and installing cabinets, a swag lamp, a refrigerator, and an oven. (In exchange for this privilege, Ms. Hart agreed to show her rooms as a model for potential move-ins. This was the only case of such extensive refurbishment that we saw in all six research sites.) Mr. Brown made the choice to sell or give away his household furniture and use what Laurel Ridge offered; he was satisfied, the sale gave him pocket money, and it eased the strain of moving on his 80-year-old cousins who helped him relocate.

Residents vary in their backgrounds, interests, health status, and family patterns. Common in Laurel Ridge is a type of family relationship known as fictive kinship, one in which relatives are defined socially, not through blood or marital ties, but instead on the basis of their actions (Schneider 1984). Mr. Sidney was not atypical in having outlived his biological relatives and his friends. "Here I am and I don't have not one single friend. All of my friends—I've outlived all of my friends, and I have. I don't have a friend that's somewhere living. You see? All of my old friends are gone. You get a funny feeling—you get a feeling, everyone—everybody—all gone. All my family—my personal family. I mean every one. . . . They're all gone." Twice married and childless, he felt "very lucky" to have been "adopted" by his second wife's family and noted that they treated him well, "just like I was one of them." Della, Mr. Sidney's great-niece, was matter-of-fact about her status as his adoptive family; she had overseen other relatives beside Mr. Sidney and expected her caregiving role to continue, pointing out that the typical African American family is much more extended than white families: "It's something you do. . . . You do what you need to do. It's not the first time . . . and it hasn't been the last time."

Joan, a fictive niece of Ms. Harriette Emory, another resident at Laurel Ridge, referred to caregiving as a "responsibility" and an "honor." "In black families, we always look after somebody." In a telephone interview, Joan had exclaimed, "Aunt Harriette was willed to me!" Mrs. Emory had been the best friend of Joan's aunt for 63 years when the aunt developed cancer. Before she died, she entreated Joan to take care of "Aunt" Harriette, whom Joan had known her entire life. Mrs. Emory's husband had long since died, and she had lost her son to a drug overdose in his thirties. Joan handled her aunt's familial, medical, and financial needs for close to 10 years, visiting at least weekly and monitoring hospice care until Aunt Harriette's death at 91. "I think it's terrible to be alone," she told us in an interview, adding, "I would want somebody to do that for me." She attributes learning her attitudes to caring and respect from her own grandmother, with whom she had been close.

Outliving the Money

Overseeing finances is the responsibility of family, including fictive kin. Mr. Sidney faced no monetary challenge, at least for the moment. Mrs. Perkins was not so lucky. She had left the employ of the federal government to open a small business. After she suffered a fall in her eighties, her husband tried to modify their home for her return, but because she was unable to use the stair chair, staying at home was not feasible. Mrs. Perkins liked the rehabilitation facility, but it was too costly. Barbara, her niece, found out about Laurel Ridge from one of its social workers. Money was tight. As Barbara told us, "We scraped and scraped and scraped and scraped." While Mrs. Perkins was adjusting to life in assisted living and, in fact, learning to walk again, her husband was becoming more frail, and Barbara was spending an inordinate amount of time running between the two homes. After a stint in a nursing facility, Mr. Perkins joined his wife. Barbara said, "Oh, boy!" "I know they didn't have that much savings," she continued. "And I said to put them up at Laurel Ridge together is going to be about $4,000 a month and—he had a little bit of money in the bank—but it wasn't that much. I said, can I get this house sold before that money runs out?"

What Barbara, Mrs. Perkins, and other residents and families soon learn is that Medicare does not pay for assisted living. Mr. Perkins' early disability and Mrs. Perkins' small business left the Perkinses with minimal Social Security benefits; this, coupled with paying for assisted living and medicines, required Barbara to take out a loan before the house was sold. She was afraid that she would have to put her aunt in a nursing home, thinking, "Oh, God, she would have a fit! . . . She's still kind of perky." In desperation, Barbara spoke to the directors at Laurel Ridge. "They said that they really don't put you in the street. I didn't know that." They told her about the spend-down program and encouraged her to apply. "I don't think they like a lot of the residents to know this." In the meantime, Barbara was asked to make funeral arrangements for her aunt. (In Maryland, assisted living residents must, at admission, state their preferred funeral home, a task approached humorously by Ms. Clinton. She envisioned a posh site in the heart of Washington, DC, hoping this would entice her artist friends to pay her a visit!) Fortunately, Mrs. Perkins' bill was reduced. "She was under the impression that the money would outlive her, you know," Barbara said, "but because longevity runs in the family, and she has such a strong will, she's outliving the money."

There are costs in addition to rent, medications, hospital and rehabilitation bills, and pocket money, which by themselves run high. Ms. Clinton spent more than $100,000 in medical expenses despite insurance before her move to Laurel Ridge. Barbara spoke of the community fee. "You have to pay a one-time resident fee in those homes, you know. . . . $2,500 . . . and so I just figured she [Mrs. Perkins] can't go anyplace else because she'd have to start all over again, and she doesn't have money to start all over again. Plus she doesn't have money to pay that initial— because, I think, any home—you have to be there a while—to spend your life savings before they try to help you out, you know." Dolores noted that the majority of families at Laurel Ridge supplement the cost of residents' care. As for moving, the payment of a community fee and eligibility for a home's spend-down program, as we see with Mrs. Perkins, work against residents who are not satisfied where they are and would like to transfer to another assisted living residence. So, too, does moving a resident's belongings, especially for older family members caring for siblings, cousins, and friends.

The Dining Room

The most sought-after and the most contentious place in Laurel Ridge was the dining room. It has a serving staff different from the care aides, whose only food-related work is to deliver and pick up people at mealtimes and help residents identified as having "special needs." The dining room was open for about 1½ hours for breakfast, and then the staff closed the doors. Afterward, the dining room theoretically was open from 11:30 a.m. until 6:30 p.m., the original design plan being that residents could eat meals at any time during the day. Despite the sign announcing these hours, the dining room closed about 1:30, allowing a few stragglers to remain, and then refused entry to residents until it opened for dinner, about 4:00 p.m. Residents complained about this, to no avail. They would line up for dinner sometimes as early as 3:00 p.m., and occasionally the doors opened at 3:30. Several of the residents could not remember when they had last eaten a meal, and they repeatedly asked the receptionist when lunch or dinner would be served. Those who entered even as "late" as 5:45 were hurried by the staff, who wanted to clear the dining room by 6:30 on the dot. If someone knew that she would be late because of a medical appointment, she could call ahead to reserve a meal.

The dining room's main entrance is off the lobby, where a sign listing the day's entrées is posted. The music that blared throughout the building, an oldies rock radio station, could be heard above the din of chatter and clanking dishes. A second door to the dining room is on a perpendicular wall which faces a hallway and the medication-cart "library." Residents would come early for supper, receive their medications, and then hang around the "library," the corridor, the TV lounge, and the reception area until the dining room opened. Those who could manage the short walk would leave their wheelchairs and walkers in the hallway, to be picked up after meals.

For most of our research tenure, four entrées a day were offered. Residents could select one entrée for lunch, then another, or the same one, for supper. The kitchen would also make sandwiches upon request, and one resident consistently had cooked cereal for many of her meals. Soup was often available, but to residents' consternation, it could arrive at any point during the meal and was rarely hot. Mr. Sidney was told by servers that he would get his soup "when he got it." There were complaints about the kitchen running out of foods of choice and about the lack of fresh vegetables and salads. Others appreciated the cook's specialties, like rice and beans and chicken wings. Because of budget cuts, only two entrées per day were offered at the end of our research at Laurel Ridge. Despite the early supper hour, evening snacks were generally not available, and many people kept food in their rooms.

At Laurel Ridge, residents could eat whatever they liked despite health problems that would dictate diet restrictions. Rebecca, the move-in coordinator, talked about autonomy in her interview:

> We can't force the residents to do anything—that's probably one of the major differences between assisted living and a nursing home. . . . We can encourage them and remind them and tell them—like, we had a resident who constantly would go out to the grocery and buy food and sweets and things like that, and lie to us. And tell us that it wasn't happening, but then when we would go and do something for them in the room, then we would find all this terrible food. And so

we would remove it and we would try and encourage them and tell them why this is wrong, but unfortunately we can't force the resident. Just like if they come downstairs—[if] they're a diabetic. . . . They go to order dessert and they want the banana cream pie, and we can say to them, "Well, it's probably not in your best interest to have that because you are a diabetic, and you know that's going to cause your sugar to go up," and they say, "I don't care. I want this banana cream pie"—we can't force them not to.

Within the dining room itself, residents sometimes had difficulty negotiating space to find a seat. Although there was no assigned seating, many residents had "their" tables and dining partners, and were reluctant to share. Four women held court in the center table, talking about everybody who lived at Laurel Ridge. Their loud speech, probably a result of deafness, made their conversations audible to almost everyone. (Mrs. Jones, not one of the four, was annoyed at what she heard.) Ms. Hart, though criticized by some, often sat by herself because she wanted to read. To Ms. Clinton, company was irrelevant; she ate wherever she could easily maneuver her motorized chair, finding more space at the close of the meal hours. Mr. Sidney, of course, ate with Mrs. Perkins.

Despite the importance of meals in residents' lives and the daily lineup to be served, we found the dining room to also be a source of conflict. Other residents took seats being saved for friends; several residents were routinely argumentative; one person periodically sang loudly during meals; a few were physically aggressive toward others in the dining room. One afternoon we found Mr. Sidney upset about what happened at lunch.

> He said he was sitting at his table and was just getting comfortable when "new people came in" and were extremely . . . "vulgar" and "profane." They were taking "God's name in vain," "screaming" at residents "something about the seating arrangements," and he found this disturbing. He said, "You lose your appetite." That day he cut our visit short. He was going to dinner early, "before a fight."

Many residents had not been exposed to the negative characteristics of dementia before moving into Laurel Ridge. Docile and quiet residents were readily accepted, and we noticed residents helping each other, from pushing a wheelchair in to a table to escorting a neighbor to his room.

The Philosophical Mr. Sidney

Mr. Sidney had a calm approach to life. He had a sense of both complacency and ambivalence, satisfied enough with his everyday existence to be accepting yet hesitant to initiate change. He felt that consistency is important in adjusting to assisted living and that learning is crucial: "You learn by doing, you know. . . . Of course, I had to ask some questions. I still have to ask questions." The "tenants," he thought, needed to make suggestions to "management." Mr. Sidney had advice for newcomers at Laurel Ridge: "People who come here have to learn to get in a set routine," and, he added, "we need to watch out for each other," just as he and Mrs. Perkins do. As he said one July afternoon, "When you've gone through nine decades, you have seen a lot, [you have] a clear view of what is going on."

During an interview a month later, Mr. Sidney spoke of what he saw when he looked back over his life. He talked about appreciating his memories. "You just enjoy it, you know. . . . You have so much experience. . . . It's really good. . . . Everyone should be able to . . . look back over things." Then he asked us to imagine how we would feel at his age. When asked "What sticks out in your mind?" he responded, "I think a lot about the people I have seen out there." Della observed that Mr. Sidney "has a beautiful way of looking at life. . . . He has a spirituality that's very real and meaningful to him. In fact, he has said on a few occasions to me that when he goes to bed at night he just asks God to—how does he put it—he asks that when he wakes up, wherever it is, it's with Him. To me, that's quite a faith. I wish I had it."

Mr. Sidney was no "Pollyanna." Della corroborated what we found in our discussions with him, that he noted and took action to moderate his decline. He watched himself deteriorate and told her, "What I could do last week, I can't do this week." Despite the daily challenges of being an old man, Mr. Sidney remained philosophical about the process of aging. "Getting old—getting old is the thing to do. Everyone should get old—that's the truth, . . . everybody should get old—if they didn't have to die—but everybody should . . . because it is good, because you look back over things."

Final Thoughts

Inclusion

Dolores would like to see a dementia care unit established as part of what Laurel Ridge could offer to potential clients, but the corporate office is not willing to invest in so extensive a remodeling. Residents complain of encountering inappropriate behavior, such as hitting, shouting, wandering, and stealing; and their tolerance levels vary, depending on the group living at Laurel Ridge at any one time. Dolores finds that families are more tolerant of people with dementia; residents, on the other hand, see those with dementia on a daily basis and become afraid that they, too, will lose their cognitive ability in the future. Some residents do feel that individuals with dementia are coddled at the expense of others, but it may be that the staff are too few and untrained to handle numerous and difficult problems.

From the nursing perspective, Joseph feels that "people with dementia really need a separate unit because it requires a unique type of care and you have to train your staff on how to manage people who have dementia. If you throw them all into the same group, it's particularly difficult because of the number of times you spend with the person who has dementia," in comparison with someone who is cognitively alert. "Wandering is something you cannot stop, but through activities you can manage that. So people have to be trained. You have to find a way for everybody." In his position as director of nursing, Joseph finds that cutting back on care aides' hours and the degree of residents' dementia are stressful on the staff, especially in regard to the care strategy of repetition. It is "the repetition of things, the refusal, the resistance to care, that's—I think that's where all the stress comes from." He also does not discount the strains of everyday "normal" assistance: "When you have fifty people to give medicine—it drains you. It drains you."

Dolores concurs: "We have a lot of behavior problems here and that takes a lot of the staff time to re-approach, re-approach, re-approach to get this person done." The charges, Dolores feels, do not reflect the amount of time direct care staff spend with residents. She sometimes tells families: "It takes us ten times—ten different people to get your Mom a bath in two days, because we're not the place where we just grab and push them and make them do it. We don't do that. But we also have to make sure that this person has a bath, and changes clothes or whatever. But sometimes we just run up against the wall." Both Joseph and Dolores feel that an enclosed dementia unit and specially trained staff would better serve all the residents at Laurel Ridge.

Rebecca, move-in coordinator and main facilitator with families and residents, takes a slightly different realistic and experiential view on the subject of a dementia care unit. "First off, I think it's a little expensive for us to look into. The other thing is that it's hard to figure out who should be in it and who shouldn't, because so many residents do stuff referred to as dementia. And we are a locked facility all over the place. So, you know, a lot of times residents who have dementia do like to walk around and roam and so . . . if the dementia facility was a wing and we locked it up, they would probably go crazy because there wouldn't be any place for them to go, for them to walk to. So, walking around here—every place is going to be safe for them to go. They can't go out."

The building is not designed for easy remodeling, and the corporate ownership is not in favor of any change, especially with Laurel Ridge's low census. However, familiarity and experience with other homes having dementia care units enable Dolores and Joseph to realize their benefit in caring for all residents. For the time being, it is easier and cheaper for the staff to tell residents to lock their apartment doors to keep out wandering neighbors. Rebecca, too, brings up a good point—the problem of confining residents once they have had the freedom to wander about the entire home.

During our research, no residents or family members complained to us about being buzzed in or out of the front door. Either it is not an issue, or it is something they are willing to accept for a good price of care. Several did note surprise at the level of dementia seen at Laurel Ridge. Mrs. Perkins said that she had never seen such people and didn't realize they even existed. Her niece Barbara "was surprised to know that they had so many patients with Alzheimer's" (often used as a catch-all for any type of dementia). She hadn't noticed this on visiting Laurel Ridge. "I didn't pick that up when I first took my aunt there. . . . I didn't realize that they had patients that didn't know where they were, until I went back to visit a couple of times, you know. And a couple of the patients started talking to me and I realized that they didn't know where they were. And now I see they're taking more and more of them up there." Mr. Sidney also was not cognizant of how dementia is manifested in residents' behavior. What he saw as conflict situations in Laurel Ridge, especially the verbal outbursts and abusive contacts in the dining room, were really behavioral issues on the part of the residents with cognitive difficulties. As Laurel Ridge continues to be census-challenged and to accept residents with increasingly more pronounced medical conditions, it will be plagued by these sources of conflict and concern.

Resident Transitioning

Laurel Ridge is similar to other assisted living homes in the area in terms of resident transitioning. As with the Chesapeake, the ages of residents span fifty years; lengths of residence vary from a few months to a decade; hospice, rehab, and respite stays are additional sources of income; some people transition to nursing homes, medical facilities, or other assisted living settings, even out of state; and a few go into independent living or to a family member's home. Some residents did see themselves as consumers. Ms. Clinton said she was "looking," but moving would have been expensive and difficult for her. "Looking" probably gave her a feeling of independence and a sense of autonomy that she lost after her fall. Within the remaining population of residents, there was relatively little shifting; people seemed content to remain in the suite into which they first moved unless there was a problem with a roommate or a private room opened up.

Over the years, Joseph has noticed a cyclical pattern. As people get physically stronger in assisted living, and as their money runs out, some move back home. They then decline because their health is not monitored and their care-giving relatives are overburdened with other familial responsibilities; he (and others) refer to this as being "sandwiched." Once elderly family members can no longer be comfortably managed at home, they return to assisted living. Then the cycle repeats.

Joseph's pattern of care highlights one example of episodic movement, as does a consumer model. In this culture, we are expected to orient ourselves to get "the best deal." Despite being consumers, assisted living residents are reticent to move. The first deal suffices for the best deal. They have already made at least one major transition, into assisted living. It is far from easy to do this multiple times. The community fee has been paid, and the resident settled in. It is burdensome to ask relatives and friends to move possessions a second or even a third time. The flexibility of Laurel Ridge to work with change in a resident's financial status and its licensing to provide level 3 care work to help residents age in place. As we saw, Mrs. Perkins used a subsidy program, and Della was grateful that her uncle, Mr. Sidney, could make use of these levels before being forced into skilled nursing.

A "dementia-inclusive" home also serves to lessen transitions. Laurel Ridge is not constrained by having to limit the number of residents with dementia, as is the Chesapeake, which has a limited number of rooms in its dementia care unit. At Laurel Ridge, the entire home is open to this type of resident, and increased fees are not applied. The residence has also designated a dining/activity room where residents with specialized needs are fed, tracked, and comforted during the day; for the night they return to suites integrated within the home.

The low census at Laurel Ridge brings about a fluctuation in direct care staff hours; the fewer the residents, the fewer staff contact hours, with staff schedules reflecting the numbers of residents, not the degree of their need. Despite this, staff turnover at Laurel Ridge is low. There are, however, latent benefits for people residing in a home with a low census. Directors, like Dolores, are often willing to broker deals to keep rooms filled. Subsidies similar to the spend-down program used by Mrs. Perkins are offered. The staff is willing to work harder with and retain problematic residents, and the home is more tolerant of negative behavior. Also, specialized needs are addressed in a myriad of ways. All of these work toward lessening resident transitioning and increasing stability in the home.

The Goal of Laurel Ridge

"Good care for a good price" is a phrase that summarizes what Laurel Ridge is all about. Mr. Sidney reminded us that "this is not a Wisconsin Avenue joint." Dolores feels that "the senior life is hard," and so she tries to lead her staff in making the final years of "her" residents' lives comfortable. "I know that I'm in this job because I care about what goes on with my seniors, period. I love them to death. Some of them get on my nerves and I know I get on their nerves, you know what I'm saying—but I'm here for their well being. If they don't like something and you can't please everybody, you know you do your best." While she feels that, ultimately, the resident has the last word, Joseph sees that care is a balancing act between what residents want and what they need. "I think you go for the best interest of the resident." He is also careful not to be "caught making decisions for the family," while Dolores leans on the side of resident choice.

Our ethnographic research at Laurel Ridge showed an unintended result stemming from caring for residents. Family members and staff spoke of residents as role models for their own old age. When I first called to interview Joan about her Aunt Harriette, she was waiting for an agent to explain long-term care insurance; she didn't want to worry her children when she got older. Caring for Mrs. Perkins made Barbara think: "Taking care of my aunt has been a lesson for me, you know, as far as preparing for my old age." Dolores, working most of her life with older people, has learned from them and visualizes her old age in assisted living. "I have had some of the best teachers. . . . I've enjoyed them, some of them have been a nightmare, but a majority have taught me how to be a resident."

EIGHT

❧ Everyday Life in Assisted Living

A colleague who heard about our study asked us, "What's a typical day like in assisted living?" The heterogeneity of people and places necessarily affects the answer. For many people who reside in assisted living facilities, a typical day might not be very different from a day spent at their previous home. They have meals, watch television, nap, read, take care of personal care needs, go shopping, work on hobbies, and visit with family and friends. Some continue to do their own housekeeping, while others are thrilled to have a housekeeper for the first time in their lives.

For others, assisted living could not be more different from home. Living in an apartment-style setting is new to many, as is having a roommate (something that a small number of our participants reported), or living in one small room as opposed to a house. For some, the daily schedule varies substantially from the one they had followed or would prefer to follow. As a result, some older adults residing in assisted living find themselves awakened or put to bed at unaccustomed times, eating meals earlier or later than they desire, or taking a shower only twice a week when they are accustomed to a daily bath. Nearly every resident receives basic services such as housekeeping, laundry, and meals, but many require help from a staff member to complete personal needs like bathing, dressing, using the toilet, moving around the residence, and taking medications. A few need almost total care. While many residents express gratitude at receiving support in myriad personal care tasks, some express annoyance at the loss of independence, resenting that they need help or that they are not given the choice to do some things on their own.

Some residents find the assisted living environment provides much more activity than their prior situations, in both positive and negative ways. Individuals who want social interaction often enjoy sharing in conversation and having something to do. Whereas the assisted living residences in our study structured their activities in the daytime, one group of women at the Chesapeake created an informal social club that met late in the evening to chat and munch on snacks. But for those who prefer privacy or solitary pursuits, the constant presence of others and the encouragement at some assisted living residences to participate in the scheduled activities (prompted by a belief that social engagement is necessary for well-being) is an annoyance. When an interviewer asked her to describe a "good day" at the Chesapeake, Mrs. Mitchell said, "Well, actually they have too many things—that you have to pick and choose. They'd have you running every single day. . . . I don't seem to have much time on my hands [for] writing notes or letters, or buying cards—and your time is taken up." This contrasts with Opal's experience at the much smaller Franciscan House, which she repeatedly described as "boring." Despite a daily timetable structured by meals and planned social activities, residents also kept to their own schedules, such as watching a favorite television show: Mrs. Koehler didn't miss *Law and Order,* and *Dr. Phil* was popular at Huntington Inn.

The preceding chapters provide in-depth stories about six residents of assisted living facilities. In this chapter we synthesize some of what we learned about everyday life in assisted living during the course of this research. In many ways, assisted living is a study in contrasts, due in part to the realities of group living. In actuality, many assisted living staff members and managers want to accommodate resident preferences, but they must also restrict some choices that residents make. Residents experience varying levels of contentment and resentment associated with life in assisted living. We observed similarities and differences across these places that went beyond the size of the facility or the type of care provided. For example, assisted living operators vary in the degree to which they are either rigid or accommodating of resident needs and preferences. Some of the contrasts and apparent contradictions we observed result from the unique perspectives of the beholder: assisted living represents different places for different people because it is simultaneously a residence, a work environment, and a regulated entity. It is a place where residents experience their own and others' illnesses and disabilities, make new friends, play card games, listen to music, and look forward to visits from family members. They receive help from workers on whom they depend for intimate personal care and medications as well as for sympathy, hugs, and jokes. To the direct care workers, the residents are the reason for their employment; some residents make the work positive and rewarding, while others, intentionally or not, are a constant source of frustration. In addition to meeting the needs of residents, the workers must also meet the demands of managers, nurses, and residents' families. Managers respond to residents, families, and staff in addition to regulatory and market forces; they are, after all, running a licensed business. Although we have less information from the perspective of people who work in the public agencies that oversee assisted living, we often heard from management and staff members about "the state" or "surveyors" who could penalize them for making errors or who make seemingly unrealistic demands. And yet, managers took diverse approaches to implementing the state's rules.

How different people in different assisted living settings respond to and manage the various elements described above results in the unique culture we observed at each place. In the following section we present some of the realities of life in assisted living, including the restrictions and accommodations and the contentment and resentment of group living. After that we summarize some of the similarities and differences across settings.

Realities of Group Living

Assisted living settings are, by design, meant to be noninstitutional (Kane and Wilson 2001), especially when compared with what might be considered traditional caregiving institutions such as hospitals and nursing homes. On many measures of institutionalization, such as physical design, professional dominance, rigid schedule, and emphasis on the group rather than the individual, assisted living succeeds in differentiating itself from traditional caregiving settings, though to varying degrees. Institutional elements are evident, however, in both the building's characteristics and the degree to which each setting is either restrictive or accommodating of individual needs and preferences.

One way in which these realities can be appreciated is in the serving and eating of food. Physically and socially, the dining room can be seen as a microcosm of the larger environment; at mealtimes, many issues, challenges, opportunities, and satisfactions are highlighted. Meals organize the day for both residents and staff members, in part because of the sheer amount of time involved in all aspects of dining: preparing food, serving it, waiting for it, eating it (or not), and talking about it on food committees and at informal gatherings like "The Forum" at Huntington Inn. Many social activities are associated with food, including celebrations and holidays that link residents to events taking place in the world outside the assisted living facility and to their prior lives. Food is also symbolic because of its connection to history, culture, religion, and family; and for these reasons, personal control and choice over what to eat, where and when, is an important topic (Savishinsky 2003).

What's for Dinner?

The smaller settings we studied were understandably more accommodating of individual likes and dislikes. At Valley Glen Home, Rani often prepared personalized dishes; one evening Nellie was having fish sticks, Rosalie had barley soup, Iveris had a crab cake, and Jane had chicken. Rani did not offer the foods typical of her native India, explaining that older people were not accustomed to the seasonings. The kitchen was centrally located in the house, with the sights, smells, and sounds of food preparation accessible to all. Throughout the day, the kitchen area might be visited by residents who liked to sit at the table for afternoon tea. And a care aide often sat there while catching up on her homework in the afternoon when residents napped. The kitchen opened onto a space that included a large table where meals were served family style.

At Franciscan House, Maria learned what foods people did and did not like when they moved in and adjusted her menu, preparing food to order as much as possible, especially at breakfast. She explained: "I have one resident who wants hard-boiled eggs every day. When you're almost 90, you can have anything you want. So whatever they want. It's not that hard. I would rather they eat. They're not asking me to bake a cake in the morning, so I say that's O.K." The kitchen was visually separate from the dining room; Maria did not encourage residents' entering the cooking space, which she kept immaculately clean. The dining room walls were decorated with Chinese watercolor paintings of pandas and Christian artwork, including a wood-carved depiction of the Last Supper.

The larger facilities tried to make up for what they couldn't individualize by offering some level of choice. Breakfast was the best meal of the day for residents at Huntington Inn because it provided the most options. Typically it would include cold or hot cereal, two or more types of bread, eggs (served to order), French toast, and pancakes. The midday meal was the largest, usually an all-in-one dish like a beef-and-noodle casserole or turkey tetrazzini. Only one choice was offered at the main meal, but residents could request cereal or a sandwich. When asked about the food, one diminutive woman said, "It's not so good but there's tons of it!"

In contrast to smaller residences, the dining rooms at the four larger settings were visually and structurally separate from their commercial kitchens. Huntington Inn had a spacious dining room, lit by expansive panels of fluorescent lights. This space doubled as an activities room; residents gathered there to make crafts, do chair exercises, and attend seasonal parties. The furniture included both large and small uncovered wooden tables, with two residents seated at each of the smaller of the tables and four to six residents at others.

The cuisine at Middlebury Manor was of the "meat and potatoes" variety. The nursing home kitchen prepared all of the food, which often was served more than an hour later than the posted mealtime, so hot items would arrive lukewarm. A typical day's main meal might include broiled chicken or slices of ham with baked sweet potatoes and cooked cabbage. Dessert might consist of a canned pear presented on a slice of iceberg lettuce or red Jell-O chilled in little glass bowls. The dining room, added when the facility expanded, reflects the existing mansion's décor. The high ceilings, windowed walls, and a gas fireplace gave the dining room a cheery look. The floor was covered in faux wood-grain linoleum. Residents kept their own assortment of condiments in the center of their bare Formica-top tables. ·

At the Chesapeake, the menu sometimes included items that were gourmet and ambitious, such as fresh rockfish and crab cakes (local specialties), saltimbocca, and crepes. Still, sometimes the kitchen staff's menu choices clashed with the expectations and experiences of the residents. When the director of dining services prepared gazpacho, the complaints about the "cold soup" that had been served were vocal and lengthy; when he served fajitas, people didn't know what to do with the tortillas. He then helped to form a committee of residents for the sole purpose of addressing food quality and menu variety. The dining room at the Chesapeake, the most elegant of the homes we studied, featured clean table linens, fresh flowers, and most notably, a grand piano. Food service was restaurant style, with a framed daily menu available at each table; individual orders were taken by the staff, and generous portions served. Despite appearances, throughout the months of our research at the Chesapeake we heard many stories about overcrowding at meals. The management revealed plans to remodel the dining room to create more space. (In fact, this did happen several weeks after we completed fieldwork.)

Laurel Ridge originally offered a choice of four entrées each day, with the menu posted on an easel just outside the dining room. To save money, the management later scaled back to two entrée choices. Residents could select one entrée for lunch, then another (or the same again) for supper. When the kitchen ran out of residents' preferred foods, the staff made sandwiches to order. We heard some complaints about the lack of nutritious foods, such as fresh vegetables and salads, but several residents also reported their appreciation for the Jamaican cook's home-made specialties, especially red beans and rice and barbecued ribs. (The staff, too, enjoyed his cooking, and one receptionist asked him to cater her sister's funeral.)

The Laurel Ridge dining room needed renovations—the dark-colored carpet had visible stains from spilled food and drinks. The executive director told us that she had attempted for years to convince the corporate office to remodel the dining room; they finally consented during the time of our study there, and we observed how the changes, including a wood floor and new table settings, improved the ambiance.

Despite differences in the sizes and configurations of these assisted living dining rooms, several of them shared common issues. Spaces became crowded with walkers and wheelchairs, making it difficult for both residents and staff members to maneuver between the tables. Residents who could negotiate the walk to their tables without support were encouraged to park their mobility aids outside the dining room. Each assisted living facility attempted to create settings that their residents would find homey and appealing, whether the country-style leanings of Middlebury Manor and Huntington Inn, the family-style dining at the small homes, or the fresh flowers and glass goblets at the Chesapeake.

Food quality and quantity were frequent topics at all these facilities. Some residents complained while others raved, yet it seemed that nearly everyone had a favorite dish or meal. Perhaps more important than the food, however, was the way in which it was served. Even though many residents, mostly women, expressed gratitude that they no longer had to cook meals each day, some missed their favorite foods and the ability to prepare it in familiar ways. Food, as well as mealtime memories, intrinsically links individuals to memories of home.

Limited Accommodations

The physical design of each assisted living residence provides certain clues about the culture of the place. What it cannot describe are the ways places are experienced by the people who use them, whether residents, staff, or occasional visitors. Residents of assisted living are there because they cannot live alone; either they need assistance to manage the activities of daily living (bathing, dressing, taking medications), or they need the safety and oversight afforded by living in this type of residential setting. Individuals, of course, have their own opinions about whether they require assistance and about how they would prefer to have it provided. For example, some residents prefer to shower in the evening, others in the morning; some want the main meal to be served at noon, others in the evening; and so on across the spectrum of daily activities. We observed that life in the assisted living setting presents restrictions and accommodations, a result of staff efforts to balance the different preferences of individual residents as well as regulatory requirements, corporate pressures, and professional standards. These competing demands mean that residents have choices but within limits.

Requirements concerning meals are among several topics included in Maryland's assisted living regulations, which mandate three daily meals served in a "common dining area" and food prepared in accordance with "state and local sanitation and safe food handling" guidelines. In addition, the regulations require a licensed dietician or nutritionist to make certain that meal plans are "nutritionally adequate." These food-related rules allow assisted living operators a great deal of flexibility as they plan and deliver food services. In addition to the state regulations, however, assisted living administrators can set "house rules" relating to food and eating.

The managers of each assisted living residence had food-related rules in addition to those described above. For example, food storage was an issue at most settings, including Huntington Inn, where one resident, Donnie, explained to us that Mr. Hill prohibited residents from bringing leftovers from the dining room to their rooms, calling it a "public health" concern. Mr. Hill argued that not only could the food attract vermin, but also that some residents might mistakenly eat spoiled food that could sicken them. (In fact, this strict house rule was the outgrowth of an episode in which a resident had placed cooked food in a cupboard.) Donnie complained that this action unfairly limited residents who could appropriately handle leftover food; she admitted to us that she occasionally hid food in a napkin and brought it to her room to eat at a later time. Mr. Hill instructed the cleaning staff to remove from each resident's apartment food that they believed to be at risk of spoiling, including fresh fruit and other snacks brought by resident's family members. Such practices, while practical in nature, left some residents questioning whose home it was, after all.

Whose Home Is It?

Each assisted living resident is a unique person with his or her own preferences and needs for a sense of home. Group living presents a challenge to some as they adapt to sharing space and daily activities like meals with others. The staff of the facilities in our study found ways to respond to these challenges by creating separate spaces for residents whose physical and psychological needs differed markedly from the others. They also resorted to measures like using assigned seating in the dining room that seemingly challenge the goal of supporting resident choice. However, practices designed to meet the needs of the larger assisted living community—such as keeping the peace in the dining room—sometimes took precedence in the balance between restriction and accommodation.

In the assisted living setting each resident has his or her own living space, in most cases a small room or apartment. For a few this space was within a shared room. To a large extent, residents personalized their own rooms with items brought from home or, for some like Dr. Catherine, with all new furnishings tailored to fit the dimensions of a 400-square-foot unit. The variety of decorating styles helped us to appreciate the differences among residents, and they shared with us stories about their lifelong collections, pictures of extended families, and items purchased during world travels. In the larger assisted living facilities, many residents spent time in their own apartments, napping, watching television, talking on the telephone, reading, or visiting with another resident or family member. Throughout the day there were many interruptions, primarily from staff members delivering clean laundry, doing housekeeping chores, administering medications, or reminding the resident about the next meal or an arranged social activity. The staff at most of these facilities had been instructed to knock before entering a resident's apartment, and for the most part this was the practice. The amount of time between the knock and the turning of the doorknob, however, was sometimes so short as to be imperceptible. The staff learned which residents were sensitive about privacy and which were not, but if a staff member felt the need to enter an apartment uninvited, he or she would do so.

Some residents grumbled about overly intrusive staff, but a more common complaint had to do with other residents—described as people who "don't belong." This category included residents whose physical health had declined to a point where they required a great deal of physical assistance and those who acted "strange" because of dementia, mental illness, or other causes. We heard comments as well as complaints about residents who dressed in strange ways, such as wearing multiple layers of clothing or patterns that did not match, and an occasional lack of clothing or public disrobing. At the Chesapeake, people complained about residents who napped in the public sitting areas—why didn't they just go to their rooms? We also learned about residents who entered others' apartments without invitation whether or not they were present, sometimes even lying down on the bed and taking a nap. Rare instances of theft were described. Mrs. Clinton reported missing food, knick-knacks, and dollar bills, attributing this to residents with dementia who wandered the halls. When told by the staff to lock her room, she reminded the assistant director that Laurel Ridge had failed to install a working lock on her door. At Huntington Inn, Frances chose to stay in her room reading or watching television rather than deal with what she described as the "gossip" among the women who regularly sat at "The Forum." She and others also complained about the smell of urine from one resident who was incontinent. But the six or seven women who regularly met to talk in The Forum described each other as friends; Karen even thought of one woman, who was 102 years old, as "like a mother." Residents regularly demonstrated tolerance toward others. One woman in this group had almost no short-term memory and was prone to wearing her slip on the outside of her dress or two different shoes. But she was also friendly, and the others simply teased her gently or guided her to her room as needed.

Occasionally, residents were disruptive in the dining room, and this upset everyone present, including the staff. Three of the residences had a segregated area for serving meals to individuals who needed extra help to eat because of physical or mental disability. The Chesapeake, Middlebury Manor, and Huntington Inn each designated a locked section of the building for individuals with dementia (or related conditions), while Laurel Ridge chose to keep those with varying levels of mental functioning integrated by placing them in apartments throughout the building. However, the management at Laurel Ridge did use a separate dining room to separate out about 10 physically frail residents who in some cases needed to be fed. In general, most facilities considered an individual who needed hands-on assistance in eating as too impaired to continue residing in assisted living. The Chesapeake required families to retain a private aide for their relative if they wanted to delay a transfer to a nursing home; some of the residents there helped blind or confused tablemates with cutting food and finding items on the table while also encouraging them to eat. Only in the small homes was it common to see a resident who needed to be fed by another person having her meal served at the same time as the others.

Some residents of the Chesapeake wondered, "Whose home is it anyway?" in response to rules about assigned seating and the meal schedule. While others might share this query, because assisted living is also a place of work and a licensed business, traditional notions of "home" become complicated. Residents might not have the final word on matters such as when to eat or who lives in the facility or whether a staff person will accompany them into the shower. Those who might prefer to manage their own medications are not permitted to do so because of the potential for harm to themselves or others.

We saw instances in which residents and staff responded in both positive and negative ways to the restrictions imposed by group living. Beyond the dining room dynamics, residents found and created a sense of home. We heard statements like "It's become my home," "Here I can choose," and "This is where I belong." When out for the day or overnight with family, many residents would comment that they looked forward to getting back "home" to the assisted living facility. Some described the other residents and staff as "like family," and we saw countless acts that indicated this was true. For example, some staff members visited hospitalized residents or came in on their days off, bringing a grandchild or a pet to visit. Residents would check on each other, genuinely concerned when a next-door neighbor missed a meal or was sent to the hospital.

In the Name of Safety

Preservation of autonomy and privacy are among the formally stated goals of assisted living, yet competing objectives such as providing for around-the-clock oversight, safety, and security, and the realities of group living can impinge on fully actualizing these values. Residents must relinquish some degree of autonomy and privacy in exchange for assistance and oversight. Most residents seem to understand the need for this trade-off; perhaps they are realists. As we observed, assisted living residences vary in how they support the values of personal autonomy and privacy in overt and subtle ways.

At each of these assisted living settings, we heard from the staff and management about the importance of the services they provided. They knew that many residents' lives depended on them, and they had examples to prove it. One of the tensions we observed and heard described related to the need to protect residents from harm while at the same time respecting them as adults. Because of concerns about safety, restrictions are imposed and enforced. Management and staff would often incorrectly blame "state regulations" when having to enforce an unpopular rule. Residents and family members more often than not would be willing to accept the restriction when the "regs" were evoked despite the fact that they were sometimes being inaccurately applied. Examples included requiring all residents to receive assistance with medications and taking a shower (at Huntington Inn), mandating that residents were not to cross the busy road to the north of the property (at the Chesapeake), requiring that the staff check on each resident at regular intervals (e.g., every two hours) through the night, and the in-room food storage restrictions described earlier.

These rules were created with the safety of individual residents and the larger assisted living community in mind. For example, the rooms at Huntington Inn did not have showers; instead, residents used one of two shower rooms that were not disabled accessible and had reportedly antiquated and difficult-to-adjust faucets. Mr. Hill insisted that a staff member be present when each resident showered, if only to adjust the water temperature or offer a steadying hand should a resident become dizzy. Although the state regulations permit capable residents to self-administer their own medications, in practice this rarely occurred. Neither Mr. Hill nor Michael Baker at Middlebury Manor (both with prior nursing home experience) believed that assisted living residents should be in charge of managing their own medications. Even if a specific resident was capable of doing so, the risks outweighed the benefits in their views: one resident could inadvertently access another's or the resident could mismanage his or her own medications. Michael told us that a major reason that people moved into assisted living in the first place was because they could not manage their medications at home. So those residents capable and motivated to manage their own medications saw concerns about safety limit their choices in these matters.

At Huntington Inn, two residents were permitted to take a shower without assistance. Each had a diagnosis of mental illness, and Mr. Hill was sympathetic to their unique anxiety about having another person present when they showered. At Middlebury Manor only one resident (out of 42) was permitted to manage his own medications. At the Chesapeake, residents who did not want a staff member to open their apartment doors to make certain they were safely in bed during the night could sign an agreement indicating that they, along with their families, accepted any harm resulting from foregoing this safety check. While these and other safety measures were an annoyance to some of the residents, others, including some family members, greatly appreciated the regular oversight.

The administration of each facility was responsible for interpreting and implementing the state's assisted living regulations. For example, the state regulations indicated that residents were to be treated with respect for their independence, choice, and privacy—that is, in line with the social model concepts described in Chapter 1. At Laurel Ridge the staff interpreted this to mean that residents could make their own choices even if a choice might result in a poor health outcome. For example, although special diets were available for residents with diabetes, if an individual chose to eat sweets, the facility would not prohibit it. Steve, the food services director, explained, "We got to give it to them." When asked why this was so, he explained that it was the "state rule" because residents were paying money and should get what they asked for "unless they can't think for themselves." Technically, Steve's comment was not accurate. State rules require that resident choice be respected, but also that facilities be responsible for maintaining the health and safety of residents—two requirements that can often come into direct conflict.

Still, the example of the "diabetic who ate sweets" is common in assisted living (Carder 2002a). It serves as an indicator of the balance between responding to residents as autonomous individuals and as "patients" in a strict institutional sense of the word. Assisted living residences are neither independent residential apartments nor nursing homes; this in-between status leaves staff, residents, and their families confused. For example, in Chapter 2 we described how Jane's daughter was willing to accept the risk of her mother's escaping through the bedroom window in order to let her have fresh air. Yet, this was not a choice Rani could allow Jane's daughter to make. At Middlebury Manor, Mrs. Koehler's daughter fought to allow her mother, who had problems managing her diabetes before moving into the facility, to stay in assisted living so that she could "die with a [television] clicker in one hand and a Bavarian cream donut in the other." And yet the daughter appreciated the medical oversight the facility provided: "Middlebury Manor has her so well regulated because they make them get up—they make them eat three meals. . . . And her blood sugar is better than it's ever been. She doesn't argue with them because they just say, this is the way it is." The administrator at this residence was proud of the facility's record of care and of the "medical model" approach he used. He explained that he hired nurses, even though not required to do so by state rules, because they were better able to meet the residents' complex needs.

The right to smoke was another topic with safety implications. None of these assisted living residences permitted residents to smoke in their apartments, but the Chesapeake had an enclosed smoking room, and the covered front porch at Huntington Inn served as the smoking area for both residents and staff. Such accommodations were important to residents who smoked, but with rights come restrictions. Dr. Smith, a resident at the Chesapeake, told us about the facility requirement that all cigarettes be stored at the front desk and distributed no more than two at a time. He said, "I resent that a little bit, because it's a bit patronizing to me—kind of treated like I was a kid or mentally defective or something." Yet, as a retired military officer, he did "enjoy the structure of this place. And it's a little bit like being in the military."

Medical Aspects of Assisted Living

Most individuals move into assisted living because of health and/or activity limitations that make living in other types of environments challenging. While assisted living is not considered a medical setting, medical services related to chronic conditions, both cognitive and physical, play a major role in daily life in these facilities. Many residents use walkers or wheelchairs, some have oxygen canisters, and others require daily monitoring of their conditions. During the months of fieldwork, we saw residents experience illnesses and injuries requiring hospitalization and rehabilitation; heard about complicated chronic conditions such as congestive heart failure, Parkinson's disease, diabetes, and Alzheimer's; and observed a few residents with terminal conditions receiving hospice care. At the Chesapeake, Laurel Ridge, and Middlebury Manor, the staff used medication carts to deliver the many prescribed pills, ointments, suppositories, and inhalers required by residents. The presence of these carts, even though they differed in style between the three settings, was an ongoing reminder that most residents had medical conditions that required treatment. Not surprisingly, the provision of health services became a focus of the daily routine, though in varying ways among the six settings we studied.

In the small homes, most residents spent the majority of their daytime hours in the living room or dining room. Rani could more easily keep an eye on her residents as she prepared meals, cleaned, did paperwork, and completed a myriad of other chores by keeping them in public view. Medications were administered, diapers were checked (but not changed), and vital signs were monitored as needed throughout the day, often in the living room.

In the larger settings, these same types of medically related activities took place in both private and public places. The tension between the social model of assisted living and the medical aspects of everyday life was an ongoing theme at the Chesapeake. The corporate office did not approve of overtly medical practices, such as administering medications to residents in the dining room, but the staff sometimes did so anyway. Middlebury Manor, with its close tie to a co-located and co-owned nursing home, took an overtly medical approach in assisted living. There, it was not uncommon to see the staff distributing medications to various residents as they sat at their dining room tables, as demonstrated by the following field note recorded about an observation in Middlebury Manor's dining room.

> Mrs. Fitzsimmons now had joined Mrs. Hoffman and Mrs. Pierson. Shortly before the food arrived, the LPN brought her notebooks and medical supplies to the table to check on Mrs. Pierson, who was diabetic. She took a sample of blood from her finger, recorded the result, and then prepared a shot of insulin, injected into her arm, or was it her stomach? I had to avert my eyes—kind of bothers me. Mrs. Fitzsimmons said she didn't think it was appetizing for them to bring around the medical waste red plastic bucket, which she had lifted to the table so Mrs. Pierson could discard the bloodied pad she held over her finger. The nurse laughed off her comment.

At Middlebury Manor the staff also kept detailed records of each resident's weight, blood pressure, and food intake and bowel movements. A relatively new resident explained the system this way: "They see that I get my medication. I guess they do that with everybody. Because see, they've got somebody who just takes care of medicine. And she sees that

I get my medicine. Sometime I get it before I come downstairs. And they take my pressure practically every day . . . they look after your medical needs. Because the other day they had one of those care takers—she's catching everybody as they came to breakfast—'Did you have a bowel movement yesterday?' I said, 'Why are they doing that?' They don't want you to have a blockage. They do something before it happens."

Another aspect of medical care concerns the people who provide the services. The majority of staff members at each setting are direct care workers, most of whom are not licensed in medical care but receive on-the-job training. The Chesapeake, Middlebury Manor, and Laurel Ridge (the three largest facilities) had licensed nurses on staff, although their duties and the physical design of spaces for medical activities differed. Staff at the Chesapeake wore uniforms of khaki pants and a collared shirt. At Middlebury Manor and Laurel Ridge, most of the direct care workers wore scrubs like those seen in some physician's offices and in hospitals. These two facilities had nurses' stations where the residents' medical records were stored; a nurse could usually be found here. In contrast, the Chesapeake's "wellness center" resembled a small corporate office. Huntington Inn took another approach, with staff dressing in casual clothing (like Mr. Hill). A tiny office, referred to as the "nurse's station" despite the lack of any licensed nurses, served as the location for storing medical records and medications. Mr. Hill had a long-term relationship with a physicians' practice, including a psychiatrist who regularly visited some of the residents; he also arranged for mobile lab services so that residents did not have to leave the building for routine lab work, including blood draws, mammograms, and heart monitoring.

The fact that many assisted living residents have one or more medical conditions, physical disabilities, and cognitive illnesses can lend an institutional feel to an assisted living setting. Yet the degree to which each setting either felt or looked like it provided medical care varied. For example, administering medications at mealtimes is convenient for busy staff and is preferred by some, though not all, residents. At Huntington Inn, on the same day the mobile X-ray technician could be seen wheeling his equipment down the hall, the woman from "mobile pets" might also be there with a friendly Weimaraner. Such scenes suggest that, though medical conditions and services occur in assisted living, they represent only part of the day.

Similarities and Differences across Settings

The culture of each assisted living setting evolves on the basis of its history, leadership, and unique pressures, as well as because of demands that are common across settings. The staff and management of a facility ultimately determine how restrictive or accommodating they will be in response to these pressures and to resident needs and preferences. These decisions significantly affect how residents experience everyday life in assisted living. As we have seen, the fact that each assisted living home serves three daily meals does not begin to describe the distinctive ways in which this task is accomplished by staff and experienced by residents.

For example, although similar activities took place at each setting, the details differed. Both the Chesapeake and Middlebury Manor had regularly scheduled lunch outings and shopping trips, as well as occasional wine and cheese socials and musical performances. At the Chesapeake, lunch outings were to bistros and upscale restaurants, while the Middlebury Manor group went to family-style restaurants. At the Chesapeake, nice varieties of wine were served in glass goblets; at Middlebury Manor the staff poured wine from a gallon jug into the same type of small plastic cups that they used at other times for dispensing medications. The many other activities common among the assisted living settings we studied—including church services, visits to the beauty salon, manicures, and monthly resident council meetings—differed just as the people living there varied in terms of social class, life experience, and expectations.

Is There a Typical Day in Assisted Living?

In trying to learn about the experiences of people who live in, visit, or work at assisted living facilities, we have largely discovered that there is no "typical day." While there certainly are structuring features, such as the provision of meals and the handling of medical and other tasks, such as personal care and housekeeping, both the ways in which facilities achieve these tasks and the everyday lives of individuals residing there are highly distinctive. The requirements of group living, including staff schedules and collective events, constrain daily routines, but there were individuals who had managed to sustain their lifelong interests and flourish in a setting that matched their needs, while others found an entirely new routine and a social context unlike their prior lives.

The "typical day" in assisted living is composed of many factors, including the many "places" that assisted living represents to the people who live, work, and visit there. Assisted living is simultaneously a residence, a business, a licensed place, and a workplace. The mix of these elements varies depending on one's role within assisted living. An assisted living residence has institutional qualities but differs from traditional caregiving institutions, in part because of the efforts of the staff to respond to residents as individuals while at the same time balancing the realities of group living. As described at the beginning of this chapter, the diversity among and within assisted living settings challenges our ability to answer the seemingly simple question, "What's a typical day like in assisted living?" Not only do the people who reside in assisted living vary in terms of their needs, life experiences, and personal preferences, but in addition, assisted living owners, managers, and employees create, through their specific approaches, places that look and feel quite different from one another. In sum, these assorted characteristics merge and form the basis of a varied everyday life in assisted living.

NINE

✿⊱ Aging in Places

···

Aging in place is frequently discussed as a key philosophical goal of assisted living. The concept broadly refers to enabling older adults to remain in their current or preferred environment, with necessary adaptations and supportive services, to the end of their lives (Bernard, Zimmerman, and Eckert 2001). The assisted living sector has adopted and adapted this concept, so, once an older adult moves into assisted living, the assumption is that he or she should be able to remain there with growing support to meet changing needs (Kane and Wilson 2001; Pastalan 1990).

The broad support for aging in place is represented in a statement by Barry, the executive director at the Chesapeake: "This is, you know, your last move (as long as you don't need skilled care), that you can pass away here with hospice just like you do at your house." A slightly different view of "place" was voiced by another Chesapeake administrator, Clare, who said that the Chesapeake encourages aging in place by having people transition from independent living to the dementia care unit. Clearly, to some residents and family "place" refers to their room or apartment, while others' views also encompass moves among multiple levels of care in the same location.

There has been a broad debate among experts about whether aging in place is a reality for people living in assisted living or whether, in fact, it even should be a goal (Chapin and Dobbs-Kepper 2001). There is also the question of whether aging in place encompasses moving within the same assisted living or continuing care retirement community setting to a different level of care—such as to a floor or building that provides care for persons with dementia, as Clare suggested. This chapter examines stability and change in the lives of older adults as they reside in assisted living facilities. We focus first on what our informants told us about the decision to move to assisted living, including how a setting is selected. We continue by discussing issues and opportunities that arise as the older person moves into an assisted living setting and remains there for some span of time. In the final section of the chapter we focus on the eventual departure from the setting, either through death or through a move to some other housing/care arrangement.

Rather than focusing on *aging in place* as a singular outcome, however, we examine the process of how aging occurs *in places,* ranging from the community (one's own home or that of a relative or friend) to assisted living residences (or varied units within the assisted living setting) to hospital/rehabilitation centers and "back home" to assisted living or to nursing homes. We also discuss the continuities and changes during these periods of residence. Relocation was the initial focus of our research project, but as we began our observations in the six settings, we discovered that the concepts of stability, change, and transition are much more complicated and nuanced than simply moving or staying in a particular place.

As a result, our discussion in this chapter addresses the many issues related to entering, staying in, and leaving assisted living, which extend far beyond the simple matters of decline and improvement in physical health and cognitive function. First, our research reinforced the well-established finding that most of the older adults living in assisted living would have preferred to remain in their own homes. Second, although the move into assisted living is often discussed as if it were a thoughtful consumer decision, our research showed that most decisions to seek housing in an assisted living facility and the selection of a setting are driven by crisis events, with limited time to consider options and with prior efforts at planning sometimes thwarted. Third, the key elements of selecting an assisted living facility focused on cost, fit, and location. A fourth transition-related finding is that many of the changes we found in the lives of older residents were managed without requiring a relocation to another setting or a higher level of care. Finally, our research also suggests that aging in place remains a complicated achievement for assisted living. For aging in place to be the right outcome, the fit between the resident's needs and preferences and the assisted living setting's ability to meet them must remain in balance through time, a difficult challenge in this dynamic environment. We learned that family, financial, and assisted living–related changes are also critically important to transitions of assisted living residents. In the end, it will become clear that "aging in place" is not necessarily to be expected, nor should it necessarily always be preferred, in assisted living.

How Is Assisted Living Viewed?

The great majority of older adults prefer to remain in their homes if possible. If relocation must occur, assisted living is viewed as substantially preferable to a nursing home. The daughter of a resident in Valley Glen, showing the extreme negativity of some in our study toward nursing homes, referred to them as the "Auschwitz of the elderly"; and another daughter of a resident there thought that if her mother "had to move into a nursing home like the one her [aunt] was in, . . . she would just die." Dr. Catherine's and Mrs. Koehler's dread of the nursing home, discussed in Chapters 5 and 6, is mirrored by that of Mr. Sidney's great-niece, who referred to them as "warehouses." Surveys for many years have consistently shown that older adults and their families fear and try to avoid nursing homes (Eckert, Morgan, and Swamy 2004). So the emergence of the assisted living sector provided an opportunity for care and support in a less medical, more consumer-driven environment (Zimmerman et al. 2003). Fortunately, there have been notable improvements in nursing homes over the years, including new efforts to change their overall culture (Thomas 2001, 2006; Weiner and Ronch 2003). Nonetheless, one would rarely expect nursing homes to be places where anyone would prefer to live, and so assisted living is expected to remain a more palatable residential care option for the future.

At the same time, assisted living is a distant second choice compared with remaining in the community and in one's home of many years or, in some cases, moving into the home of a child or a friend (Lee, Peek, and Cowart 1998). The latter preference is not universal, however; some of our respondents (and those in many surveys) clearly stated a preference to live with relatives, while others do not want to "be a burden" in the lives of their grown children or grandchildren (Lee, Peek, and Cowart 1998). For those who prefer not to move at all, or who prefer to live with family, moving to assisted living adds a disappointment with kin to the emotions accompanying the serious problems or events that require them to seek a different living arrangement. As a result, decisions about assisted living are, more often than not, stressful to both the older adult and the family.

All parties typically recognize that the move carries significance far beyond a simple residential relocation, because it signals the need for supportive services and oversight that are markers of disability and decline. In some cases fundamental aspects of one's status as an adult are threatened by entry into a group setting (such as privacy and freedom to come and go at will); and cherished daily routines (such as cooking or sleeping late) may disappear. In spite of these challenges, some older adults we studied embraced the prospect of entering assisted living, recognizing positive opportunities that included greater social involvement and a more appropriate physical environment. They also appreciated the value of services, such as meal preparation and housekeeping, as well as the physical care and support available there.

Entering Assisted Living

The Decision to Move

Few of the residents we interviewed said that they had anticipated the prospect of moving into assisted living or had sought information well in advance of need. This is not surprising because American culture discourages thinking about or preparing for disability that may appear in later life (San Antonio and Rubinstein 2004). Also, older adults and their families and friends tend to hope that they will be able to remain at home with support until the end of life. Families often delay for as long as possible conversations on this sensitive topic, which can result in stress or conflict if views should diverge. Thus, it is common for an event to force the decision, often with the added input from an authoritative professional, such as a physician, endorsing the need for greater care or a safer or more manageable environment (e.g., one with no stairs).

Most commonly, the decision to move follows a series of changes, including an individual's declining physical health or diminished memory, changes in support systems (such as the loss of a caregiver), or the development of new conditions that raise concerns about safety or well-being. After gradual decline through her eighties, Mrs. Mitchell (Chapter 6) suffered a fall that partially immobilized her. When Hurricane Isabel struck, her vulnerability alone in her house became a concern for her son. Although she attempted to age in place with in-home support from a neighbor and resisted a move to assisted living, her son finally convinced her to move. He told her: "Look, my father would not be happy with me if I left you in this house this winter. It's just not safe, and it's my job to make sure nothing happens to you—you need to do this." Mrs. Mitchell told people at the Chesapeake afterward, "Well, you know my son told me that my late husband wouldn't like it." She later accepted the move, saying, "Things sort of fell into place." Rosalie at Valley Glen is another example of gradual decline resulting in a move to assisted living. She lived in a mother-in-law apartment attached to her daughter's home but became increasingly challenged by her arthritis and cognitive decline, the first of which made it difficult to climb the stairs, and the second of which raised concerns about a variety of safety issues, such as her leaving food unattended on the stove, creating a fire risk. Rosalie's daughter made the decision that she was no longer safe and needed to move into Valley Glen, despite Rosalie's protests.

For most, an immediate crisis, such as a fall or a stroke (either punctuating a series of changes or on its own), threatened the status quo and resulted in a move to assisted living. Mrs. Koehler's story of her serious fall (described in Chapter 5) and entry into Middlebury Manor is characteristic of this sudden, dramatic change. The majority of residents we interviewed experienced a sudden crisis—a change in health, housing, finances, or family circumstance—that prompted an urgent effort to identify a new supportive care setting.

Given the events that cause the move to assisted living, the decision to move often involves input from professionals such as physicians, social workers, referral agencies, or attorneys. Physicians are often accepted as the authority in determining that an individual, in the midst of a crisis, is not able to return home. Sometimes the physician confirms suspicions held by the older adult or family members, but his or her authoritative voice often seals the decision. While some physicians are familiar with assisted living and its variations, they are perhaps more comfortable and familiar with nursing homes, which have existed for much longer. Others in the professional chain, including social workers or elder care coordinators, may provide input on how to locate, visit, and evaluate alternatives, although they may not be well-informed or helpful either. Attorneys may work with families to resolve sale of property, to finalize wills and related documents, but most especially to establish power of attorney for those with progressing cognitive impairment. Clearly, older adults lacking children or kin to undertake these duties face additional challenges in such transitions.

A Consumer Decision?

Discussions of assisted living often contrast it to nursing homes as being a "consumer-driven" sector of the housing and care market in the United States. This gives the impression that consumers effectively anticipate their need for assisted living; examine the array of options available; rationally compare the services and costs; and make thoughtful and informed decisions among the alternatives. However, as we have discussed (and as addressed in comments by Dr. Catherine's daughter in Chapter 6), this process is not feasible in the majority of cases.

Because decisions about assisted living are likely to be crisis-driven, a first move usually takes place in the context of crisis. It is necessary to make a swift selection as discharge from the hospital or rehabilitation center approaches. Often the choice is made by family members and not always with input from the prospective resident. There is little time to investigate a wide array of options, schedule multiple visits to potential facilities, and make a well-considered choice (Frank 2002). As a result, the decision is typically made with insufficient time or resources to meet the standards of the idealized "consumer model" of selecting services. Instead, there is pressure to find the best option available at the time.

The consumer model also prompts us to expect that unsatisfied customers will "vote with their feet," by simply moving to another, more attractive alternative. However, our study found only a few instances in which a consumer's preferences prompted a change to a new care setting. Despite some dissatisfaction, most people stayed.

Increasingly information is available online, including information from state agencies that regulate and monitor assisted living. But this information is often limited and cannot provide a sense of whether the place is a good fit for the individual.

In addition, there is some confusion regarding who constitutes the assisted living consumer (Carder and Hernandez 2004). In the case of Mrs. Randall, a resident of the Chesapeake, the consumer appears to have been the resident herself. Mrs. Randall noted that she had decided to move out of her home and into an assisted living residence some time after her children had recognized that living at home was hard for her. Espousing the view that living with your children belonged to the "olden days," Mrs. Randall said: "I haven't relinquished the power of attorney yet. I might have to someday, but not yet. I just want to do it myself. My children's decisions may not be my decisions."

But such autonomy as Mrs. Randall's is often not the case. Many providers instead treat family members as their primary consumers; after all, these family members are often the ones who are selecting the setting, signing the contract, managing payment for services, and contributing to care decisions. Consistent with the decline- and crisis-oriented nature of deciding about and choosing an assisted living residence, our case histories showed that typically families, not the potential resident, made the initial contact, toured the facility, and decided where and when their relatives would move. A "move-in coordinator" at Laurel Ridge said: "A lot of times what happens is, the family will come and they will take a tour and then they will decide how they feel about it. And then if they like it, they will bring their family member back and to have a look at it." That visit, according to our informant, involves families giving the older relative a "sales pitch" to convince them to adopt the place they have chosen.

In some assisted living settings, such as the Chesapeake, family members are treated as the primary consumer; they are asked to make decisions about privileges such as leaving the building, room transfers, and changes in level of care. Of course, in cases where family members have fiscal or legal authority for their relative due to dementia or other severe conditions, such primacy in decision making is expected. The Chesapeake, however, treated family members as primary consumers for all of their residents, making sure the family was provided with information about services, costs, policy changes, or other important issues. This is an interesting point, and one we will return to as we discuss fit with the setting and with other residents.

Choosing the Setting

In our study we found that three criteria were key to the choice of an assisted living facility: fit, location, and cost. By "fit," we mean that the needs and preferences of the older adult match well with what a particular assisted living setting offers (Lawton 1981; Rubinstein 1989). Residents and family members spoke to us about seeking a match between the individual and the setting on many levels, including the physical environment, the services offered, and the less tangible aspects of a setting (e.g., staff interpretation of privacy standards, the type of residents). For example, some assisted living residences have a religious affiliation either with a church or denomination or through the orientation of its owners/leaders (such as we saw at Franciscan House); this feature may appeal to some residents or their kin.

Finding a good fit is often a challenge, however. As we have seen from the diverse profiles of the settings in this study, assisted living residences offer different mixes of services, have diverse sizes and configurations of physical space, attract different types of clientele (based, e.g., on race or ethnicity, religious preference, social class, or the availability of dementia care), enact different philosophies of care, have highly variable costs, and offer distinct local cultures and amenities (such as offering barber/hair salon services or allowing residents to bring a pet). Some facilities feel like private homes, others like hospitals, and others are more akin to a hotel. One lesson that visiting assisted living settings teaches is their diversity. If you've seen one assisted living, you certainly have *not* seen them all.

For many, "fit" referred to a perception that the assisted living residence was homelike. Family members of residents from both of the small facilities in our study told us that the decision to select that particular residence was based on its atmosphere, in which residents slept in typical suburban bedrooms and passed their time in a living room with others. A family member of a Valley Glen resident explained, "I had gone to see several other ones, and it was the only facility closer to a home environment. And when I saw the loving people, I knew that was it." But that type of environment, with more limited activities and services, would not provide a good fit for some individuals. Fortunately, size does not necessarily mean a lack of homelikeness. Some residents at Middlebury Manor described it as homelike, even though it was much larger and more medically focused than Valley Glen and Franciscan House and had a physical environment that was quite different from these small facilities.

For other participants in our study, an essential factor in the assisted living decision—as it is in real estate decisions—was location, location, location. Location refers not only to the physical setting—the neighborhood and the community—but also to the proximity of one's social network, especially family and friends. At the Chesapeake as many as 50 percent of residents came from distant communities or other states to live close to an adult child. At both Huntington Inn and Middlebury Manor, the situation was quite different; many residents had lived most of their lives in the surrounding communities, and some knew the administrators, staff, or other residents personally. Thus, preferred locations typically reflect proximity to the older person's home or to that of an adult child. In the latter instances, family members sometimes expressed guilt over uprooting their parent but saw such a move as the only practical solution to enable them to provide adequate social contact and oversight.

At Laurel Ridge, which was located just outside a major city, many residents who had migrated there viewed the assisted living setting, on a busy suburban highway, as unpleasantly different from their old urban neighborhoods. They preferred their previously accessible streets and public transportation, although their physical functions had diminished so that they would not have been able to use those services had they remained in their prior communities.

Of course, other considerations also drive the choice of assisted living. Families were aware of the cost of assisted living and issues of ongoing affordability, and we frequently heard that alternatives were ruled out quickly if expenses were deemed too high. Financial realities often influenced not only where older adults moved but also (eventually) how long they could afford to stay in a particular facility. The majority of older adults or their relatives paid privately for assisted living. A small number of residents used government funds available through Medicaid waivers, which support persons eligible for nursing-home levels of care in alternative home and community-based settings.

Not only did the monthly charges vary among settings, but so did the way fees were categorized and presented to the consumer. In some cases, the charges were bundled so that housing, meals, and services provided for a given level of care were quoted as a single monthly figure. Elsewhere some services, such as assistance with mobility or for incontinence supplies, were "a la carte." Some assisted living facilities charged fees such as the "community fee," which was nonrefundable after a certain length of residency.[1] In these cases, there was an established basic fee for room and board, and then a menu system to select additional services. In this second model monthly costs were variable and, to some extent, not predictable. In most cases a premium was charged for more intensively staffed dementia care services, whether these residents lived in the general resident population or in a separate unit.

In setting their fees, assisted living providers were well aware of the local markets, the likely competitors, and the growing awareness among consumers of alternatives, such as bringing services into the home. The administrators clearly understood that they were running a business. The administrator of Middlebury Manor said: "We can't change the physical plant. So this building—and it's not, it's not as nice as newer facilities are . . . very nice facilities. . . . So really our niche is to get—to really focus and get back to our niche—is to get back to being the lower-cost provider." Those assisted living residences that were challenged to keep their rooms filled sometimes were more flexible in terms of fees. Both Middlebury Manor and Laurel Ridge struggled to fill their rooms and were willing to negotiate service rates. In fact, Middlebury Manor marketed itself as a lower-cost provider, more affordable than other nearby facilities. As a way to manage its costs, this facility arranged, through informal risk agreements, for family members to provide some services there, such as changing bandages or assisting a relative with bathing.

Perhaps above all, the choice of an assisted living facility (especially under time pressure) depends on whether or not a preferred provider has space available. Some of the residences in our study consistently had waiting lists—sometimes long ones. In these cases, families might not be able to wait until the facility that was their first choice had space available. Mrs. Drake entered the Chesapeake at a time she considered "too early" because she was encouraged by her daughter to act so that she would not "lose her spot." But waiting lists can often be deceptive, because invariably some on the list will have been forced to select another assisted living residence by the time a vacancy occurs. And some marketing personnel as well as concerned family members have been known to exaggerate the difficulty of obtaining a room, creating a sense of urgency to encourage the older adult to make the decision sooner.

How Do People Get Information about Assisted Living Facilities?

Older adults and their family members learn about assisted living options through formal channels as well as by informal communication with others in the community. Some assisted living settings, especially small ones, are "hidden in plain sight," despite being located on busy streets. That is, they lack outward signs of being a specialized housing setting and so do not build public awareness by making their presence obvious. At the other extreme, Laurel Ridge posted a sign outside the building, along a busy road, promoting its reduced monthly rates.

Many of those we interviewed reported that they began their searches with official lists from local agencies or offices on aging. Experts in health or community service settings also made referrals. For example, workers at local hospitals referred some of the individuals we profiled to residences with which they were familiar. Several Laurel Ridge residents told us that this home had been suggested by physicians at the Veterans' Administration hospital where they had been treated. Daughters of two residents on whom we focused, one at Valley Glen and another at the Chesapeake, had hired elder care consultants, who provided information and tailored their suggestions to settings most likely to be responsive to the specific needs of these older adults.

Despite these formal sources of information, referral by word of mouth was the most common way that residents and families learned about assisted living settings in their communities. Many interviewees recounted stories of either an older relative or a friend who had spent time in a particular facility. The family members of one resident told us that they learned about Middlebury Manor from friends who were "in a similar situation with their aging parents." Also, clergy and religiously based social services groups, while not expert in assisted living, had referred a number of residents to Laurel Ridge, based on their familiarity with it.

Referrals were important to the assisted living facilities. Marketing was a major concern for some (but not all) in our study. To market Laurel Ridge, its directors visited area hospitals for referrals and developed rapport with the hospital staff. They also visited skilled nursing facilities, anticipating that there might be occasions when patients there would be discharged to assisted living. The objective of the staff person responsible for marketing at Laurel Ridge was to keep her assisted living residence "alive in the community." She visited local doctors' offices, community centers, and churches, giving gifts and providing lunches. She felt that some of her best referrals came from the people she met during coffee hours in church on Sunday mornings.

The Chesapeake, part of a large chain, maintained a nearly full resident census on the strength of its desirable location and reputation, paired with active marketing in the community. The managers at both Huntington Inn and Middlebury Manor reported not needing to advertise much, relying instead on the development of informal referral networks in the community. Other assisted living settings in our study struggled to maintain occupancy rates about 70 percent of capacity but could not afford slick marketing materials or staff time to do significant outreach.

Things That Cannot Be Known before Moving into an Assisted Living Residence

Despite significant efforts on the part of those visiting and considering alternative assisted living residences, certain aspects of life and care cannot be known until one spends considerable time, as a resident or a visitor, in each setting. Several factors that may be important are difficult to gauge from an outsider's perspective.

Fit with the Setting and with Other Residents

Even though a good "fit" is one of the criteria on which the choice of an assisted living residence is made, pre-move visits (or "tours," as the marketing staff say) seldom provide families the opportunity to learn whether the space, philosophy, services, and social environment will suit their relative. A visit may not reveal whether there is a commonality in residents' social traits, such as social class, religion or political views, or whether the privacy practices or activity levels meet individual needs. Some places, such as the Chesapeake, encourage the involvement of all residents in planned activities; this expectation may suit some residents but not all. For example, we encountered complaints that activities were too female-oriented, a criticism that the Chesapeake tried to address with a men's group. As Dr. Smith reported, "One time Richard took four or five of us [men] out to lunch. And I thought it was going to be a fairly frequent occurrence, but that was it. It never happened again."

Visits to the assisted living facility prior to move-in may provide a sense of more or less activity than is the daily norm. Many people suggest that multiple visits, including some that are unannounced, will be more informative as to whether the setting will suit the tastes, as well as meet the needs, of the person who may come to reside there.

Another experience that cannot be evaluated ahead of time is the impact of living in the same facility with persons with dementia. Cognitively intact residents and their families rarely know what it is like to live with people with dementia. Some facilities minimize this issue by having separate units for those with dementia, but people with diminished cognitive abilities are common in the general assisted living resident population (Morgan, Gruber-Baldini, and Magaziner 2001). In Laurel Ridge, where the high-functioning and the cognitively impaired residents were completely mingled within the setting, the benefits and challenges of having such neighbors can be learned only after living there. Mrs. Perkins claims not to have known that such people even existed before moving to Laurel Ridge!

Of course, given that the new resident is often moving after a period of declining health or an acute event or crisis, few residents visit the assisted living setting before moving. Family members are left to make these visits and weigh the alternatives, typically with their relative's preferences clearly in mind. When it became apparent that Mr. Wilson could not stay in his home, his son found Laurel Ridge. Several residents said they had seen the facility in which they now resided or knew of it before arriving, having worked or lived nearby or driven past it in their communities, but had never been inside until the day they moved.

In judging fit, there are also situations in which the family's preferences might not be the same as those of the prospective resident. The Chesapeake treated family members as primary consumers and asked them to make judgments for the residents. Families tend to more highly value aspects such as safety, while residents value privacy and autonomy. Mrs. Hatcher became angry when the staff of the Chesapeake removed a chair she had pushed under the doorknob to prevent the staff from entering her room during the night. Although it seemed to our ethnographer that Mrs. Hatcher was capable of making this decision, her family could and did override her choice. In cases when values come into conflict, we wonder whose "fit" is actually being considered.

Fit with a setting can change over time, making what was initially an excellent choice less optimal. While we typically think about an individual's progressing dementia or increasing medical needs as challenges to be considered when choosing a facility, the assisted living residence itself may also change in ways that reduce fit. A change in ownership, the addition of a dementia care unit, or turnover of leadership or key staff may result in significant alterations in the setting, services, or cost that drive a decision to seek care elsewhere. Nellie at Valley Glen had arrived there after several prior care experiences, including one in a setting that was sold to a management firm that failed to make key repairs to ensure safety and health.

In some of the settings we studied, greater flexibility in the approach to care enabled even people with terminal illnesses to remain in their assisted living "homes" with support from the area hospice organization. Field notes from the Chesapeake record the comments of a tearful son who, mistaking our researcher for a member of the assisted living staff, expressed his thanks "for letting his mother die in the way she wanted." She wanted "to stay out of the hospital and die at home," which is how she referred to the Chesapeake. Such flexibility (or its absence) may not be apparent during an initial tour.

Leadership and Staff

It is difficult to gauge certain intangibles of attitude and orientation toward care in a typical visit to an assisted living residence. Our research found that there are marked differences in settings, even in those that are part of chains, based on the style and approach of their managers. The style and philosophy of leadership also shapes the composition and priorities of the staff members who create the daily experience of assisted living residents. Fit with direct care staff is perhaps the most salient component of what it feels like to live in a given assisted living home. These staff members provide 90 percent of the direct care to residents and are the ones who have first-hand knowledge of when change occurs (Stone 2000).

The view of administrators, enacted through care staff in daily routines, influences the tone and feel of a setting (Mead et al. 2005). Some family members interviewed at Valley Glen, an unassuming small home, expressed gratitude for the ability of one administrator to provide such loving care in her small environment: "I think it is partly that she picks [staff] people who are decent, but I think it is also that she is an incredible role model, and they get into it." Other family members of residents at Valley Glen talked about the administrator's role and its importance to the stability of the residence. In a place like Valley Glen where the administrator is the owner, there is no less concern about a turnover of leadership changing the nature of the setting. In other settings, we witnessed frequent leadership turnover, sometimes resulting in significant change.

Mr. Hill, the owner-operator of Huntington Inn, died suddenly during our research there, and Mrs. Hill hired a person known to the couple who had experience as a nursing home administrator. This new administrator immediately changed the orientation of the facility. Huntington Inn quickly came to take on the routine and feel of a nursing home. Both residents and staff were dissatisfied, with several members of each group leaving during this administrator's brief tenure. She was replaced by a manager also known to the family who shared their philosophy of care. When an arrangement with the second administrator to purchase the facility from the family fell through, a young woman who had worked her way up through the ranks at Huntington Inn as Mr. Hill's assistant director took on the job as administrator and continued the philosophy and approach to care that was familiar to both residents and staff.

Long-Term Cost

Residents and families frequently voiced concerns about the cost of assisted living, especially in the context of not knowing the duration for which assisted living services would be needed. Although prices and charges are disclosed when a person enters assisted living, providers sometimes change their fees or the way that they charge for their services.

Facilities with flat rates based on one's "level of care" can change to a menu-based approach. Over the duration of a stay in an assisted living facility these changes, along with increased costs driven by changes in residents' health and functioning, can result in quicker spending of limited resources. Mrs. Jackson was cautioned by an attorney before entering Middlebury Manor to ask what would happen if her money ran out. Despite having saved for her old age, because she was now spending about $3,000 per month, she said, "My money's going to run out pretty soon." In many interviews, both family and residents expressed worry about whether the money would hold out long enough to enable the person to age in place.

Moving and "Settling In"

Transitions into assisted living were not always straightforward or linear. For one resident at Laurel Ridge seven months elapsed from the time she first left her house for the hospital until she finally settled in the assisted living residence; her entry was delayed by an interval of rehabilitation, two falls, and deferral for treatment of an infection.

It should come as no surprise, then, that through our work we discovered that the settling-in process varies for each individual. Responses from both staff and residents to questions about how long it takes a new resident to settle in ranged from no time to several months—or even up to one year, in the eyes of the Chesapeake director. Similarly, reactions of new residents varied widely, with some adjusting to their new surroundings with little apparent difficulty. For others, however, the move was traumatic and highly emotional.

In part, how one reacts to such a move and adjusts upon arrival is shaped by life history, personality, attitude, and expectations. Having interests and activities that could be maintained after the move (such as in the arts, religion, or the stock market) facilitated the transition, to the extent that health and resources permitted their continued pursuit. Several women at Middlebury Manor continued an interest in needlework; at the Chesapeake Dr. Smith constructed model airplanes; and Mrs. Clinton at Laurel Ridge catalogued her many paintings and prepared to resume her artwork. Many residents still attended church with family members or fellow parishioners.

Obviously, people do not change their core orientations to life, their likes and dislikes, or their interests and goals when they become residents of an assisted living home. It is the responsibility of the facility's staff to learn about each resident as an individual, and, when residents have dementia, to get information from family or friends to help convey this individuality. Several of the assisted living residences in our study asked families to complete life history forms to inform the staff about some of these details. Without such knowledge, the staff cannot provide person-centered care, which is an important component of good-quality care.

Residents' family members are also important in the settling-in process. Some staff members complained that too often residents were just dropped off their first day. They claimed that family members did not help with the unpacking or provide moral support as their relative dealt with the complex meaning of the move. On the other hand, from the perspective of family members, these moves—and often the accompanying closing down of the parent's household—were accomplished with significant tangible and emotional effort on their parts. Doubtless there is a range of family support from high to low through this transition because some families are emotionally close and local while others are emotionally or geographically distant.

One area in which families are commonly involved is the downsizing that must occur when a family member is moving from a house or an apartment into a smaller assisted living unit. Another is dealing with the related financial and legal transactions. Belongings are reduced to little more than bare essentials, and furniture and real estate may need to be sold (Ekerdt et al. 2004). Along with disposing of belongings and property, family members may also be engaged in attempting to establish eligibility for Medicaid waiver funding, dealing with insurers, and gaining power of attorney, all the while continuing to attend to their own daily jobs and relationships with their own children and grandchildren. Mrs. Koehler's story is one of several reflecting these combined challenges.

The administrators and staff of the various settings facilitate residents' adjustments in a variety of ways. Rani, the manager at Valley Glen, focused a great deal of time and attention on her new residents, cooking their favorite foods to make them feel at home. Maria at Franciscan House concentrated on ensuring that the new residents' medical needs were being met and on helping them to integrate into her stable daily routine. Mr. Hill showed the new residents the dining room and presumably introduced them to others during meals. The manager at Laurel Ridge recognized the need for a social worker to help in this settling-in process but was unable to add one to the staff because of the necessity to minimize staff costs.

The importance of getting to know other residents early in the settling-in process was viewed as important. In fact, some managers and staff members discouraged family visits early during the transition, to encourage the new arrival to interact with others and begin to engage with activities and staff on site. Dr. Catherine's daughter (Chapter 6) indicated that she cut back on shared meals with her mother, "trying to help her get, you know, interact with people there. And that seems to be sort of their first way of meeting each other is through their table companions."

Many times, other residents were helpful in assisting with transitions and adjustments —after all, they had been through them before. The residents at Middlebury Manor created an informal welcoming committee, volunteering to introduce incoming residents and show them around the facility. The administrator of Middlebury Manor recognized the need for this group; while the committee was never made official, the administrator relied on and encouraged the residents' informal efforts to ease in newcomers.

Obviously "settling in" is a highly individual matter, with definitions of what it means varying widely. The attitudes of those first moving into an assisted living facility vary from anger and sadness to acceptance and optimism. These individuals have to learn to live in a new physical environment, with a new set of peers whose circumstances, interests, and actions may conform to or differ greatly from their own. They also may need to adapt to a new daily routine, new smells, and new noises. Paired with whatever circumstances prompted the move, these demands may be a significant stressor on an older adult.

Despite this potentially difficult transition, newly arrived residents experienced varied reactions. Some continued along their trajectory of physical or cognitive decline. Other individuals went through periods of anger or depression, and still others faced accelerated decline in their functioning. This was often the case for those with dementia, who typically found the unfamiliar environment and new routines highly confusing for a period of time.

Not all of the residents had negative reactions. Some experienced improvements in their psychological and physical well-being after settling into the new environment; after all, assisted living was intended to supply them with needed support. Those who had lacked desired social contact found new friends, as did Mr. Sidney and Mrs. Perkins, or expanded social networks. Still others benefited from regular health evaluations, regular receipt of their prescribed medications, and oversight of appetite and other markers of potential health problems, as well as the removal of the demands of home maintenance and meal preparation.

Creating a personalized environment by hanging photographs on the wall, placing belongings on a bookshelf or windowsill, and bringing furnishings from one's previous home are a few ways in which settling in takes place. In nearly all of the rooms we visited we saw family photos and other personal items that gave the feeling of a homelike environment. In facilities that accepted them, small pets also made the setting more familiar. Many of these personal touches were often present in the rooms of individuals with dementia, despite the fact that they might not recall the identities of all of the people in the photos or, poignantly, that those depicted were no longer living.

Once a Resident: The Complexities of Change while Aging in Place

How Long Do Residents Stay?

One question frequently asked by researchers, policymakers, and consumers of assisted living services is how long residents remain in any given setting. Our study was not designed to provide statistical estimates, but other studies have shown that on average the older adult who moves into assisted living will remain there less than 3 years, with stays ranging from very short term, due to planned rehabilitation, death, health decline, or immediate dissatisfaction, to an exceptional few residents who remain for many years (Hawes, Phillips, and Rose 2000; Phillips et al. 2003). Thus, some individuals reside in an assisted living facility for years with relative stability in health, fiscal, and familial status.

However, the more common pattern over an extended time is a continuation of the decline in mental and physical health that initially brought the person to assisted living—or the development of new problems. The potential for stability, most particularly in how well the environment fits a resident's preferences and needs, is shaped by the reality that older persons in assisted living typically have severe chronic health or progressive conditions, such as problems of mobility or dementia. For example, earlier research showed that more than half of residents in assisted living settings from four states used devices to support mobility, and the average resident had limitations in two of six areas of daily life (e.g., getting in or out of bed, eating, bathing, and mobility) (Morgan, Gruber-Baldini, and Magaziner 2001).

Staying or Moving: The Tip of the Iceberg in Understanding Change

When we began our research, we were interested in residential transitions of assisted living residents, specifically moves into and out of assisted living. This narrow point of view quickly broadened to examine how individuals in assisted living experience stability and the multiple types of changes in their lives during their stays. Most of these changes, rather than prompting relocation, result in some adaptation on the part of the person, the family, or the assisted living setting. So our research quickly expanded beyond the study of staying or moving to include many elements of the unfolding dynamics of residents, staff, and facilities in assisted living.

Changes we observed were of numerous types and degrees of importance. They included acute health episodes (such as falls or facility-wide flu outbreaks) that required residents to visit hospitals or necessitated restrictions on visiting; residents' changing rooms within the facility due to events such as renovations, the establishment of a new dementia care unit, financial challenges, or health needs; changes in the ownership or administration of the assisted living facility, with potential changes in services and approach to care; turnover of direct care staff; and changes in family support and involvement in the care of the resident or oversight of services (due to death in the family, an employment-driven relocation, or shifts in family relationships). The most common change was in a resident's health or functioning, including decreased mobility, problems related to medications, or the emergence of new health conditions to compound those already present (Ball et al. 2004).

One key lesson we learned is that care facilities can absorb numerous changes without residents' having to relocate to another assisted living facility or to a nursing home. The changes may, however, alter the fit between the needs of the older adult and the physical environment or services of the residence. In such an instance, aging in place may not be in the individual's best interest. As we saw in Chapter 4, Mr. Hill, the owner of Huntington Inn, defined personal mobility as important and required that residents be able to get themselves to the dining room for meals. Although other rules were flexibly enforced, limited staffing necessitated that residents be self-sufficient in this manner. In that setting, mobility, including use of a walker or wheelchair, was a pivotal element of aging in place.

Again, residents and their kin sometimes avoided thinking about the potential next step in the housing and care trajectory. For example, Terry, the daughter of a resident at Franciscan House, said, "I'm a planner, believe me. I plan everything." But in terms of where her mother might need to go next, Terry confessed, "I'm not even going to think about it until it happens."

The Social Interpretation of Change

Stability and aging in place were the goals of those residents who enjoyed their assisted living home, or who worried about a move to a potentially less desirable alternative. As one resident said of her future, "I'm here for good!" But the determination of whether or not a resident could remain in the current environment did not rest on the resident's or family's choice alone. Ongoing evaluation of residents' status by family, staff, physicians, and administrators fundamentally influenced how a particular change was interpreted. Some changes could be managed, allowing aging in place, while others, including those that crossed particular thresholds such as the mobility standard at Huntington Inn, might require relocation.

This chapter has already discussed some factors, such as financial or facility changes, that may prompt moves. Of particular interest to us was the more interpretive process that occurred in determining whether a change in a resident was meaningful—that is, whether it had reached a particular threshold where some action was required in response. Often the action considered was a move to another setting. As a case in point, by Maryland regulation, each resident's medical status should be evaluated by a licensed nurse every 45 days. This evaluation does not always occur as scheduled, but it is intended to determine the person's designated level of care. Even this process was somewhat interpretive, for we observed distinct differences between residents designated at a similar level within or across facilities. It was sometimes difficult to understand why some residents were transferred to a nursing home while others remained in the assisted living setting. It is not clear whether and to what extent the need to maintain sufficient occupancy to sustain staffing or profitability, having "favorite" residents, or other subtle considerations helped to determine outcomes of changes relative to relocation decisions and resulted in inconsistencies in how the rules were enacted.

Even apart from regulations, the staff and directors convey messages about changes in health or behaviors to each other and to family members, sometimes using value-laden labels. For example, the staff at Middlebury Manor referred to Mrs. Koehler as "nursing home material," indicating their assessment that her care needs had moved beyond what the assisted living setting could or should provide. While such comments may sound negative, they suggest that staff members are aware of behaviors or problems, such as repeated hospitalizations or falls, that serve as "red flags" that the person's functioning no longer fits with the level of medical services or staffing provided in the assisted living setting. In such cases, the level of acceptable risk, the capacity to bring additional services to bear, and financial matters all may shape when—and whether—a relocation is completed.

Staff members sometimes showed more flexibility in their assessments when care could continue to meet a resident's need despite decline. One woman with dementia at Huntington Inn (dubbed "Mother" by the staff because she carried a baby doll) was sometimes disruptive in the eyes of others living there, but she was not required to move into the secured dementia care unit. The staff seemed to like "Mother" and did not press her family to change her room, even though other residents who seemed similarly impaired were required to move to the specialized unit. It did seem that residents who were favorites of the staff, especially some who had been there many years, may have benefited from greater flexibility in the interpretation of rules.

The concerns about whether changes will lead to relocation, probably to a less desirable circumstance such as a nursing home, may lead residents to try to cover up health conditions or progressing dementia that might trigger such a feared change. Whether hiding deteriorating health conditions or problematic behaviors places anyone at significantly greater risk is an important question that remains unanswered.

Departures from Assisted Living

While we saw instances of moves from one setting to another to seek a better "fit" to the resident's needs, to lower costs, or to seek higher-quality services, most of the residents on whom this study focused, once settled, remained in place for a span of time. Inertia, familiarity, fear of moving to a less desirable setting, the stress of the move, community fees, convenient location, or satisfaction with the setting meant that moving as a consumer choice to another assisted living was infrequent. We have already discussed a number of reasons prompting departures, including erosion of fit due to changes in a resident's physical and cognitive functioning (changes that required more medical services or supervision), the search for a setting that provided desired amenities or services, preferences of family members, or reactions to the quality of the environment. In some instances departures are initiated by the consumers—either the residents themselves or their family members—while others are prompted by the facility's perceptions about its capacity to provide appropriate care and meet the person's changing needs. Assisted living settings vary widely in the criteria (both the assisted living facility's rules and those mandated by states) for requiring residents to leave due to level-of-care needs, specific medical care concerns, or behavioral problems (Hawes et al. 2003).

Regardless of the fit between the resident and the facility, there is always an eventual departure from assisted living—even if the departure involves a hospice-supported death in the setting. In some views, other types of departures from assisted living might be deemed as "failures," most specifically failures to age in place. Our research suggests that leaving is much more complicated, in that there are multiple types of departures and diverse stories of how and why a resident moves out of a particular place. Thus, while it is tempting to view resident departures as an indication of "consumer choice," most moves out of assisted living are not necessarily the residents' choice.

First, departures result from death following chronic illness or an acute event, which would by some definitions constitute having successfully aged in place. Death accounts for the departure of approximately 15 percent of assisted living residents each year, including those cases where residence in assisted living lasted until a final hospitalization was required or hospice care was needed (Zimmerman et al. 2005b). Ambulances taking someone to the hospital are a familiar sight at assisted living facilities, and in some cases, these trips will be the final departure from assisted living.

Another approximately 15 to 20 percent of assisted living residents leave their current setting each year, typically for more health-care-oriented settings, such as nursing homes (Zimmerman et al. 2005b). Such moves are prompted either by a health emergency or by the recognition and gradual decision that adequate care and medical services can no longer be provided to the resident in the assisted living setting. In some cases, moves to a nursing home occur because the resident has run out of money to pay for assisted living care and are driven by eligibility for Medicaid after personal resources are spent down.

While not within the control of the consumer or provider, state rules and policies also play a role in determining when departures occur. Some states require that residents who need skilled nursing care be discharged from assisted living, and others allow residents who are dying to remain there only if hospice care, delivered by an outside agency, is in place (Mollica, Johnson-Lamarche, and O'Keeffe 2005).

Avoiding a Departure from Assisted Living—When Possible

The issue of cost as a factor in departures was raised earlier. We learned that several of the assisted living facilities in our study quietly worked with residents who were running short of money to maximize the length of their stay. In some cases, a family member could hire care aides privately or undertake certain chores, such as laundry, to minimize costs at the assisted living setting. Middlebury Manor would move residents to smaller rooms without a private bath or to the adjacent nursing home (on Medicaid) when their money ran out. The Chesapeake offered a small church-funded stipend to a few individuals. Because Laurel Ridge typically had less than full occupancy, it offered 10 percent of its open rooms to people with low income at reduced rates. It did this through an in-house subsidy referred to as the "Pastoral Fund" because clergy were so active in the history and daily life of the residence. The executive director said: "It's good for the community, it's good for the resident—why leave an open bed, when you can get some amount of money?"

Laurel Ridge declined to use the Medicaid waiver program in favor of the Pastoral Fund, a decision supported by the facility's corporate office. Some other assisted living settings did use the state's Medicaid waiver program, which had a limited number of slots available for people in assisted living. Longtime residents at Laurel Ridge also had facility support to remain if they had "spent down" their funds over many years of residency there. Mr. Hill at Huntington Inn was adept in working with residents to help them become eligible for the state waiver, advising them and their relatives regarding the related policies and procedures. Smaller assisted living residences typically had few resources other than Medicaid and adjusting their fees to assist residents to finance their care.

Is Aging in Place in Assisted Living a Reality?

The ideal of aging in place has mixed support among the facilities where we conducted our research. Several of the assisted living settings aspired to provide aging in place by expanding services (sometimes from a menu at increased cost) or embracing the use of hospice within their regular operations. In other cases, managers or corporate offices identified assisted living as one step along a theoretical "continuum of care"; thus, moving individuals along to a higher level of care as their capacities declined is based on policy. The director at the Chesapeake told us that the staff at this facility begin discussing with relatives the need to move a resident to their dementia care unit in advance of the move, as soon as early signs appear. In some cases this eventually escalated to threats of discharge in the face of extreme family resistance. The staff there also prepare the family member for the move and the increased cost of specialized care. Elsewhere this process might prompt a search for the next setting for care, whether another assisted living residence or a nursing home. As noted above, there is a risk that signs of decline or diminished functioning might be hidden by some residents and families who do not wish to move (or to pay more).

Beyond differences in how facilities approach the aging in place issue, there lies the more fundamental question from earlier in the chapter: Is aging in place always the most desirable outcome for assisted living providers or residents? In our study we learned that assisted living homes, as well as their residents, experience significant changes over time. Turnover of leadership, changes in corporate ownership, or shifts in the mix of residents over time may make a particular setting a poorer fit for a particular resident even if he or she has not experienced significant change. While we typically think of the changes that erode fit as those occurring in residents' physical or cognitive functioning, the settings themselves provide an additional dynamic that can dramatically alter the fit between person and environment in a positive or negative way.

Because needs of residents, aspects of the assisted living facility, or both change through time, the outcome may be significantly diminished fit. Residents or their kin may become less satisfied with the setting, the providers may be incapable of meeting a resident's needs, or both may recognize the need for a change. Nellie, whom we interviewed at Valley Glen, had experienced a dramatic decline in the quality of care and services in another assisted living facility when it was sold to new owners. We expect that Valley Glen's environment and routines changed when Rani decided to nearly double the number of rooms by constructing an addition to her small home after our research concluded there. We have already recounted the upheaval that occurred at Huntington Inn after Mr. Hill died and was replaced by a manager from the world of nursing homes.

With few exceptions, the assisted living sector developed to provide services to older adults whose needs were limited and primarily nonmedical. Early developers learned that initial fit with the environment could easily erode over time as residents aged in place. They had to adjust their services accordingly or ask residents to leave. As primarily for-profit businesses, most assisted living providers have no choice other than to be concerned about the fiscal bottom line; thus, they are left to balance their clientele's growing needs for care with the cost of these services. Decisions about keeping a resident—permitting aging in place—are sometimes driven by concerns other than the preferences of their resident and family consumers.

On the opposite side of the equation, increasing services often translates into increasing costs, which are ultimately borne by the consumer. When this is the case, some individuals have no choice other than to seek a lower-cost alternative, and a significant proportion worry about what will happen once their money runs out. Further, if residents remain in these settings as they continue to decline, it becomes unclear how and to what extent they would ultimately differ from nursing home residents.

So, rather than being a somewhat idealized philosophical issue, aging in place as an outcome and a value runs into real-world constraints from many sides. Some of the assisted living administrators we interviewed in this study indicated that they believed that assisted living was moving in the direction of being more like nursing homes as the health of current residents declined, as newly admitted residents entered with poorer functioning, and as states' regulatory standards were developing in directions reminiscent of those for nursing homes. Certainly the future of this philosophical goal for assisted living settings is questioned more broadly today than a decade ago.

Aging in Places

We have learned from our research in these six assisted living settings that aging occurs in places. While many people do live out their remaining years in assisted living, with intermittent hospital stays, temporary residence in a nursing home, or rehabilitation visits along the way to a final illness, other residents find it necessary to move to a higher level of care (often a nursing home). Another subset will move through several settings, sometimes ones that are quite different—including some moves back home— as their needs change or their facilities change in ways that reduce fit or satisfaction.

Many dynamics, both personal and those related to the physical and social setting, can and do influence whether a person thrives, stabilizes, or declines when he or she first arrives at assisted living and over subsequent months or years of residency; these same dynamics shape whether the particular assisted living setting meets a given resident's needs or preferences regarding critical issues such as privacy and opportunities for social engagement. The challenge to residents and their families is to recognize and react to dynamics of change and to monitor the quality of fit over time to ensure that the setting, given available alternatives and constraints, is the best possible match for the resident. For many older adults, aging in place has, for now, been supplanted by aging in places as our society and economy continue the search for new models of how to provide flexibility, autonomy, and personalization in housing and care for older adults in balance with conflicting goals such as safety and oversight.

TEN

❀ The Reality and the Promise of Assisted Living

A ssisted living communities are an important element of the long-term care continuum, with more than a million residents and 38,000 to 68,000 facilities as of 2006 (NCAL 2007). Lost in these numbers is any insight into the lived reality and promise of life inside these settings. The findings from this in-depth ethnographic study allow a sustained view of the assisted living experience, providing an opportunity for better understanding by consumers, their families, providers, policymakers, researchers, students, and others interested in this type of housing and care. In addition, looking inside the walls gives a view of challenges and opportunities that make up the future of assisted living.

The first half of this chapter describes eight core realities of assisted living that emerged across the group of settings we studied. The second section considers the promise and future of assisted living as informed by this research. That future is shaped and constrained by both internal and external factors, such as the "success" of having residents age in place, the policy and regulatory environment, potentially shifting consumer care preferences, funding and financing limits, and workforce challenges clearly already at the doorstep of this relatively new option in long-term care.

The Core Realities of Assisted Living

Heterogeneity

A common refrain among those familiar with assisted living is that "once you've seen one assisted living setting, you've seen one assisted living setting." Some commentators complain about the lack of uniformity (Bruce 2006; Carlson 2005), primarily because, unlike the standardization of the highly regulated nursing home sector, it allows for variations in both quality and range of services. They argue that this variability makes it more difficult to monitor whether dependent older adults are receiving the care they need and the services they desire. Focusing on consumers, proponents of universal standards for assisted living argue that the heterogeneity creates unfair challenges for residents and their families: locating a facility in one's own community, much less in another state, is too complicated. Given that the move into assisted living often occurs during a health or social crisis, comparison shopping might not be possible, yet the heterogeneity of assisted living residences demands spending time to find the right place. Further, medical professionals and others who work on behalf of older persons might not understand that one assisted living residence, for example, accepts persons with dementia, while another does not.

Other experts, however, see the range of environments, prices, service packages, and amenities as a natural response to diverse consumer demand and as exactly what the concept of assisted living was intended to provide. If assisted living operators are to provide a setting that is "homelike," then it would follow that the wide range of what constitutes "home" in the broader community would be true as well in long-term care. Thus, for some, Valley Glen Home meets the standard of home, while for others the choice would be either the Chesapeake or Laurel Ridge. As demonstrated in earlier chapters, the diverse settings in the single state we studied vary in their structural and organizational characteristics and in the lived culture of that home for all who participate in its days and nights.

We selected our six settings to reflect key structural and organizational elements identified in other research and policy reports. These elements include the size of the facility; its for-profit or nonprofit status; its urban, suburban, or rural location; the services and amenities it offers; and the socioeconomic and sociodemographic characteristics of the residents served. For example, all of the residences studied here are categorized as "for-profit," yet this designation masks the significant differences between the small "mom-and-pop" operations (with six or eight residents) and the larger corporately owned and operated chains. In these larger assisted living residences, the structural and organizational characteristics are more bureaucratic and hierarchical, with formal differentiation of staff roles (e.g., direct care providers, housekeepers, food services) and "shift work." As organizations, the larger residences share more traits with nursing homes, from which the assisted living sector tries hard to distance itself. To some people the for-profit designation of the various settings we studied implies benefits to the assisted living owner at the expense of the resident consumer; such a perspective belies the ethic of service which we found in some of these for-profit care settings (Morgan, Eckert, and Lyon 1995). Some of the owners and operators we interviewed describe how good-quality care has an impact on the bottom line and contend that profitability is tied to their reputations as providers of high-quality services.

The structural elements described above are only a framework within which the assisted living culture emerges. One clear example of the importance of culture that we observed was how the concept of assisted living and the stated philosophy of each operator, corporation, or owner translated into daily life and routines. In examining the marketing materials of the assisted living residences in the study, we often found statements of their intentions for how services would be provided. These philosophies, however, were not always enacted with the same consistency. The key role of administrators within the organization in managing facilities, staff, and services often determined whether a philosophy was enacted or discarded.

The importance of the administrator in assisted living culture was illustrated by the change in leadership at the Huntington Inn (Chapter 4), where the owner's philosophy of making staff needs a priority had led to low turnover, creating an established culture comfortable to both the workers and the residents. Following Mr. Hill's untimely death, his replacement immediately instituted changes that led to staff dissatisfaction and turnover and to the relocation of a number of the residents, who no longer found the setting to be to their liking. Nothing structural about the place or its stated mission had changed—yet everything had changed. Similarly, a facility serving primarily those with dementia will differ from one serving older adults with primarily physical challenges or one where those two groups mingle (as at Laurel Ridge), even if their structures, sizes, and missions are the same. One cannot assume that assisted living facilities are standardized in the way that nursing homes, subject to national regulations, have been.

This concept of an assisted living culture may also explain what people "feel" about a particular assisted living residence when they walk inside. It was common for our ethnographers, researchers from other studies, and prospective residents and their families (who had less experience from which to make comparisons) to have a sense of how "good" a facility would be shortly after walking through the door. From quick observation of residents and staff, seeing the nature of their interactions (or the absence of such interactions), and smells, sounds, and other elements, we formulate a sense of the place that goes beyond size, activity schedule, meal alternatives, cost, and range of services. Whether or not this initial feeling is borne out over time is another matter. But it does reflect the fact that the culture of a setting—the everyday experience of living and working there—is more than the bricks and mortar, the dimensions of a room or apartment, and the organization.

Dynamic Lives within Dynamic Environments

Residents and their families, direct care providers, and administrative staff experience change in three ways. First, there are changes driven by time, as people evolve within the setting. Residents age and their health and well-being may be affected, families become more familiar with assisted living routines but may face challenges in their own lives, and staff members become more or less skilled or motivated in the performance of their jobs. Second, people come in and out in the course of a day. Staff members present during the day may not be present in the evening, and families who visit in the evening or on weekends may not be aware of routines and dynamics during the day or during the work week. Third, members of these various groups also exit the setting. Residents die; staff members and administrators leave for other jobs or retire. In short, while the walls may look the same, a consistent dynamic flow of persons into and out of the facility may also contribute to a changing culture.

The influence of an assisted living facility's size on aspects of culture and life for residents, staff, and others in the setting remains a point of interest. We might expect that changes would be felt more profoundly in smaller settings, where any one individual has a larger impact on the others there. For instance, the death of one resident among five might be more profound than a death would be in a setting with 65 or more residents. However, when viewed from the inside, the changes in any one person—resident, staff, or family—can have a profound impact on others. For residents, staff turnover, the loss or gain of a friend in the setting, and the availability of support from kin and others may all make a substantial difference in quality of life and care. A larger setting allows for more numerous interpersonal contacts, and so such alterations may ripple among individuals to touch more people's lives. Or, alternately, the change may be buffered by the presence of so many others. Once again, there is no sure way to predict how changes will affect the local culture as perceived by insiders; what is sure is that such change will be felt.

The Consumer Process versus Crisis Decisions

In the ideal world of assisted living, decisions about the care of an older adult are planned with full information, consideration of a range of appropriate choices, and sufficient time to weigh the relative costs and benefits of alternatives. But as we have seen, such an ideal consumer-oriented process is not typical. Our interviews with residents and family members indicate that the decisions to move into assisted living and then to select a facility tended to be event-driven. As a consequence, choices were limited to what was available in the vicinity at that particular moment and by the amount of time that could be allocated to collecting materials, visiting facilities, and comparing alternatives.

Similarly, many of the changes that require a decision once the adult is in assisted living, such as whether or not a resident needs to be hospitalized, occur quickly. A few, including those involving relocation to a dementia care unit or to a higher level of care, sometimes provide enough time to plan, although as we saw in Dr. Catherine's case (Chapter 6), even knowing that specialized dementia care will be needed does not mean that all parties will agree on the timing. Assisted living is a setting in which the staff are familiar with the events that drive various crises, the steps that must be taken to remedy the specific problem, and many of the alternatives that would be appropriate. Clearly, a trip to the hospital or quarantine for an outbreak of flu needs to happen quickly, requiring immediate decisions based on previous challenges with residents. In such circumstances, the medical model of care in assisted living overrides the social model of care; individual preferences and autonomy must be placed on hold to respond to the perceived best interests of the resident.

Negotiating Aging in Place

As discussed elsewhere in this book, aging in place was one of the great promises of assisted living when it began. Originally, leaders and advocates promoted an implicit promise that once someone moved into an assisted living residence, he or she could remain there until death. Today this promise cannot always be kept. The reasons are many. Operators recognize that there are limits to the services that some assisted living settings can provide due to staffing, physical setting (e.g., disabled accessibility), or state regulation. Older persons might prefer to move to a nursing home to receive a higher level of medical care and supervision. Health care and social service providers weigh in on whether or not specific individuals can or should remain in a given assisted living residence, and these individuals do not always see eye to eye. For example, as we saw in Chapter 5, during one of several nursing home stays, Mrs. Koehler's own doctor did not believe that she needed ongoing skilled nursing care, but the medical director at the nursing home disagreed.

Enacting aging in place has turned out to be a highly variable process, presenting challenges for those inside assisted living. Declines in a resident's health over time raise questions of whether doing so is possible or even desirable. Consequently, what arises is a dynamic situation wherein an individual's changing needs and (frequently) desire to stay confront the ability or willingness of facility management to be of help. The resulting situation is often a negotiation entered into by parties who have at their core the same basic interest: the well-being of the resident. The question remains how much assisted living should be expected to do in terms of medical services, end-of-life care and other services extending into the terrain that was traditionally claimed by nursing homes.

Despite their heterogeneity, many assisted living settings share a broad, common definition that distinguishes them from nursing homes. That definition, espoused in state regulations and by trade associations, characterizes them as providing a social model of care, designed to support residents' independence, dignity, privacy, and choice. Although facilities vary in how explicitly they communicate their philosophy among employees and in their marketing materials, nearly all providers readily acknowledge that they have no desire to transform their settings into nursing homes. Nonetheless, the distinction between the two is in flux. Our study identified many instances where residents' independence, dignity, privacy and choice were not always respected when challenging health or cognitive needs arose. Further blurring the line between nursing homes and assisted living, movements are under way to bring "culture change" into nursing homes. Such changes include patient-directed care and buildings designed to be more homelike (Thomas 2001, 2006; Weiner and Ronch 2003). At the time of this writing, Maryland, like some other states, does not require assisted living residences to have a licensed nurse on staff, although many facilities do, and others contract with a nurse as needed.

Another critical difference between assisted living settings and nursing homes is in regard to who pays and who regulates. In assisted living today most financing is private, coming from residents' funds or from relatives or through arrangements such as the Pastoral Fund at Laurel Ridge. Nursing home care, in comparison, is available to any U.S. citizen who needs that type of care and meets the financial eligibility guidelines— that is, nursing home care is a public entitlement. Because of this, standardization and regulation focuses on the care settings where the highest percentage of total costs are being covered by Medicaid funds from federal and state (public) sources—i.e., nursing homes. Given that Medicaid is a health-based program, the focus of nursing homes on the medical aspects of residents' care should not be surprising. Some assisted living settings accept Medicaid payment on behalf of residents who qualify for that program, but the Medicaid agency, the Centers for Medicare and Medicaid Services (CMS), permits states to define and regulate assisted living, including safety and quality standards. For these (and other) reasons, the level and type of oversight required of assisted living settings pales in comparison to that of nursing homes.

Residents and staff members view assisted living as a superior alternative to the nursing home for all except those who need ongoing skilled nursing care. As we have learned, determining who needs skilled nursing, and at what point in their health trajectory, is a complex and sometimes idiosyncratic process. In some cases the need and timing are clear, while in others, the decision of the administrator or medical personnel to transfer or not to transfer a resident can seem arbitrary. For example, Mrs. Koehler (Chapter 5) was able to move from the adjacent nursing home back to assisted living because of her personal relationship with the owner's family, according to her daughter. In other instances, as we've described, moves to the nursing home are a consequence of running out of funds rather than health changes. Still other residents are transferred to nursing homes from assisted living because they have complex medical care needs.

People Matter: Assisted Living Is Highly Interpersonal

Assisted living is fundamentally a people-oriented service business, in which a resident or the resident's family exchanges payment for room, board, and care. The six care settings we have described in this book demonstrate the variety and complexity of the relationships among the residents and between the residents and the workers and senior staff members who care for them and assist them in negotiating their lives and needs. In smaller settings, such as Valley Glen Home or Franciscan House, the personal relationships that develop between residents and their caregivers can sometimes be described as quasifamilial. For example, the ethnographer's note describing the care taken in braiding Miss Helen's hair in Chapter 2 shows the underlying personal connection between resident and caregiver; describing such actions as merely "grooming" belies the emotional bond witnessed here.

The story of "Mother" at the Huntington Inn in Chapter 4 shows how special feelings of affection among staff members toward a confused resident who wandered out of the building and fought with other residents prevented the administrator from moving her to the locked dementia care unit. At this assisted living residence we also observed close relationships among a group of female residents who humorously referred to themselves as The Forum. Within the larger facilities we observed greater gender diversity and the formation of "couples" between men and women sharing common interests. Thus, we found the social and relational world of assisted living to be rich and diverse. Elements of a successful social environment included a friendly and dedicated staff and a population of residents who were compatible in background and mental acuity.

Fit Matters: Person to Environment

How well a particular individual fits in with other residents and with the staff in the setting, and how well compensatory services serve particular people, is an important and continually negotiated process throughout each individual's stay in assisted living. We discussed the evolving nature of residents' fit with their environments in Chapter 9. We found that it is not only residents who change: we were astonished at the ongoing developments in some settings, including turnover of staff and leadership, changes to the physical environment or its uses, change of ownership, and alteration of the philosophy of care. Consequently, negotiating and sustaining the fit between a person and a setting is more challenging than simply addressing the resident's health status or situation at any given time.

We might argue that the diversity and the absence of standardization in assisted living facilities today serve to support negotiations of people and place by providing choices intended to meet diverse needs and preferences—in short, to maximize fit. In some cases, and up to a point, personal relationships can serve as a buffer against change. In others, fit erodes to the point where the assisted living facility, physicians, family members, or some combination of these groups drive a move to a new care setting—another assisted living facility, care at home, or the nursing home.

Business Matters: Assisted Living Is a Business

Whether it is small or large, rural or urban, an assisted living residence must be viewed as a business, based on consumers (either the resident or a family member) purchasing room, board, and care services from a vendor. Whether the assisted living facility is a profit or nonprofit business, and whether it is motivated by a mission to help older adults and/or the bottom line, its managers must hire staff members, maintain the physical plant, and take in sufficient profits to continue offering services. In the larger corporately owned and operated settings, stakeholders extend to investors who expect financial gain. Thus, a core element of assisted living is who pays and from what revenue sources.

Overwhelmingly, assisted living is financed through private funds from its consumers. Among our six settings, however, the funding sources varied. In four of the assisted living settings, people eligible for Medicaid waivers were accepted, although waiver "slots" for assisted living placement were in short supply. (The waiver is described on page 229, note 2.) In the two settings that did not accept Medicaid, other privately funded subsidy programs or accommodations were in place to assist a limited number of current residents who were running low on funds. As illustrated by two of the focal cases, and by many other residents we met, finances affect older persons' ability to move into or remain in assisted living. Such alternatives provide some "cushion" to the current occupants of assisted living, softening the business aspects slightly, but not resolving the larger issue of affordability, which will be discussed later in the chapter.

For managers, expenses for facilities, food, and, most important, staffing must constantly be weighed against revenues, which in most cases derive from the monthly fees (packaged or à la carte) collected from residents. Empty rooms or units reduce the assisted living owner's income; such losses must be balanced while new residents are sought to fill those vacancies. On the other side of the equation, families report the stress of managing and preserving money to keep a parent in place and of sometimes having to add their own money to a pension or having to use the profit from the sale of a home to fill a gap. Often families are also monitoring or paying their parent's bills for assisted living and other expenses, such as medical services, and providing for necessities such as transportation to medical appointments, clothing and toiletries, medications, and personal supplies, including those for hobbies and interests.

The challenge of being a successful business is perhaps greatest for operators of small homes, where one person or a couple must be responsible for all the tasks of providing direct care to residents, planning and preparing food, overseeing the staff and facilities, and maintaining relations with family members, as well as performing all of the necessary business duties. While the operators of the two small assisted living residences in this study managed most of these duties themselves, doing so clearly was demanding. In our view, they thought of what they did in terms of a mission to help others and support their families, not as a profit center. Nonetheless, the bottom line had to matter.

The Promise: Challenges and Opportunities in Assisted Living

We end this view inside assisted living by looking forward. As this relatively young sector is maturing, new challenges arise and existing ones continue. Indicative of this ongoing process is the fact that a federally established working group failed to generate a definition for assisted living that all participants could endorse (ALW 2003). We continue to lack a societal consensus on what assisted living is or what it should be.

Challenges and opportunities for providers include the dynamic policy and regulatory context, dilemmas arising from the success of aging in place, the critical role of sustaining a high-quality workforce, and the constantly shifting preferences of consumers regarding how, and where, to receive services in later life. Later in this section, we discuss the ongoing challenges to consumers, which include assisted living affordability and accessibility and the ongoing difficulties of understanding options and making decisions within such a dynamic and diverse sector.

The Dynamic Policy and Regulatory Context

As we have already seen, in every state assisted living moved quickly from a nonregulated sector to one having some degree of regulation. No federal regulations currently exist. But even the current state regulations, deemed insufficient by some experts, have added significant new responsibilities for inspections, care planning and reporting, which perhaps weigh most heavily on small assisted living residences with limited staff. State, county, and local governmental regulations set the stage on which the reality of life in assisted living is enacted, with periodic inspections by entities as diverse as the fire marshal and health department. This regulatory context is dynamic within the current system; how regulations will expand in the future is unknown.

Our research revealed that current assisted living regulations are in flux. Managers reported that the emphasis placed on aspects of their operation by state regulators varies from year to year. One year assisted living residences might be responding to an emphasis on food and nutritional issues (e.g., are menus posted and refrigerators cold enough?), and the next year the focus may be facility control of over-the-counter medications used by residents. As a result, inspections were cause for anxiety among assisted living managers, a fact that was sometimes noticeable to residents and their families. Among the smaller residences in Maryland, state regulations were often seen as a burden, taking up valuable time that would be better spent serving residents' needs.

In the next several years, the type and extent of regulations placed on assisted living will be influential in how this care setting develops relative to other alternatives. It remains unclear whether today's limited state regulation will persist in light of the inevitable occurrence of negative events, especially as assisted living populations become older and frailer, and percentages of residents with dementia climb. A common governmental response to a negative event is to attempt to address it through regulations, an approach that can never prevent all possible bad outcomes when applied to such a vulnerable population.

Two regulations under discussion in Maryland as our study concluded in 2006 would require "awake overnight staff" and the hiring of a full-time nurse. It is believed that these requirements, clearly more easily met in larger assisted living settings and nursing homes, would help prevent bad things from happening to residents. But they are also likely to have unexpected outcomes, such as significantly increasing the costs for housing and care and moving the assisted living option beyond the reach of some potential consumers or more rapidly depleting resources for others. Some residences that are now operating on a shoestring might even be forced to close. This pressure to try to regulate away risk can be seen as moving assisted living much closer to nursing homes in terms of the autonomy and choices that might be available to residents.

The Success of Aging in Place: Is Assisted Living Becoming the New Nursing Home?

Pressures beyond those of regulation have been pushing the assisted living sector toward looking and feeling more like nursing homes, especially those of a few decades ago. When it was a new option, assisted living attracted residents who had arrived at the point in their lives where a decision about housing and care was required. They chose assisted living on the assumption that they would age in place, with additional services to meet growing needs. Since then, both assisted living residences and nursing homes have experienced an increase in the severity of physical and cognitive problems among their residents. The move to the nursing home (possibly from an assisted living residence) happens later in an individual's trajectory of health problems, when he or she is sicker. Assisted living settings receive requests to allow residents to stay as long as possible, so they, too, house people with more problems requiring support and medical care. In short, some of the appeal to consumers and providers that fueled the rapid, initial development of assisted living as an alternative to a nursing home has been muted by the challenge of successfully enabling residents to age in place. Some commentators say that assisted living residents look like nursing home residents of 10–20 years ago. Whether that is a positive or a problematic outcome is debatable.

Based on our study of six different settings, we conclude that assisted living is resisting becoming the new nursing home, at least in terms of the regulatory requirements that define the contemporary nursing home. While in many cases assisted living residents look like nursing home residents, assisted living settings today remain free to vary how they address needs and preferences, offer services, and select amenities. But there are limits to what assisted living facilities are willing and able to provide within state regulations, and there are risks of litigation should something go wrong. Some bring in hospice to provide additional care and sustain residents to the end of life (as with Karen in Chapter 4), but others mandate that when residents reach an end point that is distinct, they must move to a higher level of care. Home operators must constantly weigh their risks, resources, and options and, in some cases, convey the bad news that "Mom must go."

Finding motivated people already involved in providing assisted living is fairly simple: many operators of facilities and many members of their direct care staffs work there because of the rewards of helping others and because of a love for older people. It is also simple to locate individuals for whom this work is "just a job, just a paycheck," and not a lucrative one in many cases. One of the major concerns we heard from operators of assisted living facilities is the ongoing effort to find, train, and retain the "right" staff. Studies over many years have shown uncomfortably high rates of worker turnover in long-term care, and assisted living is no exception. We observed considerable turnover at all levels during the fieldwork for this study and took note of problematic staff members being terminated. But there were also individuals who had been doing this work for many years.

Providing direct care to older adults can be physically and psychologically demanding and typically is poorly paid. Some bosses expect—and get—the worst from their employees, from absenteeism to an "it's not my job" attitude toward their work. Given the key role direct care staff and other staff play in the overall quality of life and care in assisted living (Zimmerman et al. 2005b), finding employees who discover sufficient rewards in the work to counterbalance its demands remains the goal. Raising pay might help in recruitment, but that would be mirrored by rising costs for care, and potentially fewer people residing in assisted living; consequently, directors or operators walk a fine line attempting to find strategies that maximize retention of good people. Mr. Hill at Huntington Inn (Chapter 4) told us that, in some ways, the needs of the staff come first because the needs of the residents cannot be met without good staff.

The workforce challenge in assisted living is only a subset of the larger societal issue of finding and appropriately training enough individuals to meet the needs that will unfold over the next few decades as the cohorts of the baby boom move into later life. Assisted living vies for workers with nursing homes, home care agencies, and hospitals, all of which require staff to provide daily care and support to their clientele. Some point to immigrant workers to meet this need; others focus on effective use of technology to help fill the gap. But the reality is that well-motivated people are required for assisted living facilities to remain in business.

Shifting Consumer Preferences and Options

Assisted living is no longer the shiny new option among long-term care alternatives. As this approach to elder care has matured, many other options for senior housing with service have been developed, including Green Houses (Thomas 2006), intentional or co-housing communities where groups of like-minded individuals create their own version of senior housing (Yeoman and Peebles 2006), and "naturally occurring retirement communities" (or NORCs) with added support services (NORC Public Policy 2007). These and other new programs have developed to meet the needs of adults who want to age in place within their current, or an alternative, community. Just as assisted living was once a hot new concept, these options are now discussed with enthusiasm and seen as providing even more varied alternatives for the coming baby boomers. Another recent growth area, active adult communities, will also present interesting questions as their "active" population becomes less so with the passage of time.

Clearly, what develops next will be driven by consumer preferences, which can be hard to predict. But preferences are typically moderated by cost, so the alternatives will also be shaped by either personal finances, as has been the case for assisted living, or public funding, as has been central with nursing homes. Some of the above options attempt to minimize costs through using or developing interpersonal networks of reciprocity, substituting for family bonds to provide care and support when these are unavailable. But ultimately, both the marketplace and preferences may create numerous or few additional competitors for the existing nursing homes and assisted living residences of recent decades.

Funding and Financing Care: The Affordability of Assisted Living

Today's system of care in assisted living is not available to everyone. It is most accessible to those who can afford to pay privately, either from their own savings or, more rarely, through a private long-term-care insurance package. The system has a major gap for moderate- or low-income individuals, who may vie for limited state or other subsidy funding but will otherwise be priced out of even considering assisted living care. Currently, their choices include care by family or friends or, if they are eligible, a bed in a nursing home, funded by Medicaid. Given the tight economies of assisted living residences and the fact that they need to generate profits while keeping prices at a competitive level, it is hard to see how relying on the marketplace will generate alternatives for "affordable assisted living," although several innovative programs are attempting to do just that (Pynoos, Feldman, and Ahrens 2004).

In their interviews with us, both family members and residents made clear that the cost and affordability of the assisted living residence was a strong determinant of their choices, and they hoped to avoid a future move driven purely by running out of money. Moving for financial reasons was an outcome to be avoided if possible. The cost of assisted living care can dip into the resources of adult children, diminishing their own nest eggs for retirement and for their own future care needs as well. Some of these family members told us that they were considering purchasing private long-term-care insurance so that they would be financially prepared should they ever need assisted living.

The Challenge of Being an Assisted Living Consumer

Whether we are speaking of the residents or the family members as consumers, occupying that role remains a challenge. Diversity among assisted living settings, while useful in finding a good fit, nonetheless means that each place you consider provides a different type of space, range of services, social environment, and cost, including differences in how the cost is calculated (what's included, what's extra). Trying to sort through this complexity in finding the best solution for yourself or a relative is challenging and difficult. Both concrete and intangible elements seem to go into these decisions, but the transition is fraught with considerable anxiety, including wondering whether you have made the right choice.

Even after the decision is made, the consumer role within assisted living is somewhat different from being a consumer at a store. If a consumer is dissatisfied with assisted living, he or she must consider that complaining may create ill will from staff members or administrators that could lead to unfavorable reactions in the future, especially if, for example, there is a desire for the resident to age in place. And, unlike returning a faulty camera to the store, it is challenging to find an alternative if a resident wishes to "vote with her feet" by moving. Concerns regarding the alternative setting may raise questions as to whether that older adult is going to have a better outcome in a new place. On balance, the bulk of those we interviewed, residents and their family members alike, were pleased with the current assisted living setting and often expressed wishes to remain there.

Conclusions

Over the past two decades, assisted living has become an important housing and care option for older adults and their families. At its best, it is an innovative, high-quality long-term care option for people who otherwise might move to a nursing home. At its worst, it faces those challenges that are all too familiar from agencies and settings dealing with vulnerable populations of all ages.

Realizing the issues and challenges that arise as older adults age in place within assisted living, a variety of advocacy and policy-oriented groups have arisen to represent consumer, industry, and policy interests.[1] However, the positions of these groups are not all alike. Some promote stronger consumer protection for assisted living, others focus more on "best practices" for those providing assisted living services, and still others push for standardization of assisted living, an outcome challenging the "consumer-driven" notion of the early days of assisted living's development as a sector. These groups join the advocacy, policy, and provider organizations that have existed for nursing homes and other specialized housing and care settings serving older adults.

As assisted living matures as a sector, we see facilities facing challenges unanticipated by those who started the field: growing levels of health and cognitive impairment among residents, issues of managing costs in the face of growing service expectations, and maintaining an identity distinct from the nursing home as consumers, residents, and some advocates push to expand options for aging in place. Clearly, pressures exist to find ways to offer affordable assisted living for those who lack the resources to pay for market-rate assisted living residences and yet do not want to receive care in a nursing home. In short, the current system, while offering options, remains a system in flux and one in which the consumer remains highly challenged to make choices within a dynamic environment. Thus, in our view, assisted living is an emerging phenomenon in step with the evolving needs and demands of aging consumers in need of housing and care. It is not without challenges. We believe that as aging boomers increasingly confront personal needs for housing and care, the drum beat for consumer protections and oversight will become louder even though the current rhythm of personal and societal values for individual choice and autonomy will intensify. In the end, we believe that some version (or versions) of assisted living will remain among the options and innovations in caring for older adults.

Technical Description of the Research Project

··

This appendix describes in detail the qualitative research process that informed this book. Our study, entitled "Transitions from Assisted Living: Sociocultural Aspects" and funded by the National Institute on Aging, was designed to provide an understanding of the minor and major life transitions experienced by residents in assisted living. Using ethnographic methods, the research team studied daily life in six settings, exploring interactions among residents, their family members, direct care staff, and administrators. Data in the form of in-depth interviews and field notes, collected between 2001 and 2007, provide the core ethnographic material to help us understand not only the topic of transitions from assisted living but also the culture of this type of long-term care. Ethnography offers a perspective different from, but not antithetical to, traditional survey research; it thus contributes to and enhances our detailed knowledge of life inside assisted living.

Research Design
Research Objectives

The main objective of this study was to understand the social and cultural factors that led to transfers into and out of assisted living settings. The specific aims of the research were the following:

1   to examine the social and cultural processes of change and decline leading to transfer from assisted living;

2   to explore how residents, their families, and the assisted living staff observe and talk about signs of decline, improvement, normalcy, and change in residents within the social and cultural environment of assisted living;

3 to understand how the local explanatory models used by residents, family, caregiving staff, and administrators influence the processes of stability, decline, and change and how they relate to decisions about retention and transfer;

4 to examine how facility-level characteristics shape the processes of stability, decline, and change.

Our ethnographic research used the qualitative methods of participant observation, intensive interviewing, and extended focal case study to better understand daily life inside assisted living, particularly from the perspectives of the individuals residing there. The basic research design consisted of sequential ethnographies, lasting 6 to 10 months each, in six diverse assisted living settings in Maryland. Following the Collaborative Studies of Long-Term Care (CS-LTC) typology, we conducted ethnographic studies in two small, two traditional, and two new-model settings (Zimmerman, Sloane, and Eckert 2001). We also collected performance-based physical and cognitive assessment data on strength, capacity to walk, and response to standardized cognitive questions with a sample of residents. In addition, during the time of our investigations the state agency responsible for overseeing assisted living facilities began a two-year series of public meetings on assisted living regulations, and a member of our research team attended many of them.

Ethnography

Ethnography involves research on individuals and groups within their own sociocultural and/or physical environments—the places where they live or work. Information is collected primarily through participant observation and in-depth interviewing. By immersing himself or herself in the setting, the researcher is able to both observe and participate in daily activities (hence the term "participant observation") and thereby comes to understand the nature and meaning of interactions and ideas through the eyes of those who live and work in a specific place. In-depth interviews, conducted in an open format, provide essential information from the perspective of the individuals being studied, including their daily lived experiences and the processes involved in formal and informal decision making. The resulting data consist of interview transcripts and ethnographers' descriptive and interpretive notes recorded in the field. In qualitative research, significance is determined not through statistical analysis but through the interpretation of events and interactions and the identification of common themes and patterns.

Confidentiality of Information

Before we began our study we sought and received permission from the assisted living administrators to observe and interview in each setting. We sent letters to residents and their families informing them of the project and offering the right of refusal to participate in the research. We obtained verbal consent from every person we interviewed, with that consent typically audiotaped at the start of the interview. In the book, we have used pseudonyms for persons and assisted living facilities, and we have altered certain details of both the assisted living settings and the persons interviewed to protect the identities of those involved. All research participants are protected by the confidentiality standards under the Institutional Review Board (IRB) of the University of Maryland, Baltimore County, as directed by the National Institutes of Health.

Selecting Research Sites

Assisted Living in Maryland

Assisted living settings in Maryland include both small and large homes (housing as few as one or two residents and as many as 150 or more) operated by both for-profit and nonprofit providers. Residents range from the formerly homeless to the affluent and from individuals who require minimal supervision to others who are eligible for nursing home care. Assisted living monthly charges ranged from as low as $400 per month to more than $6,000 monthly at the time of our study. Maryland is one of a handful of states that uses the phrase "assisted living" as an "umbrella" category to include a broad range of settings that in other states might be called "adult foster care," "board and care," and/or "residential care." Some states, and the major industry trade groups, use a more delimited definition that requires licensed settings to provide disabled-accessible apartment units (with private bathroom and kitchenette) and to follow a "social model" of care (Mollica, Johnson-Lamarche, and O'Keeffe 2005).

In 1996, Maryland officials reclassified small board-and-care homes under their new "assisted living program" regulations; before that time, homes with two to four residents had the option of being "registered," and larger homes were operated under county and state health department oversight but were not licensed (Morgan, Eckert, and Lyon 1995). The state's assisted living regulations were implemented in 1999 and revised in 2004. Proposed changes at the time this book was being written suggested revising the definition of assisted living to include three classifications based on level of care, with homes that are licensed at the highest level required to employ registered nurses (OHCQ 2005).

Selecting Research Sites

The goal in selecting research sites for this study was to identify settings that represented a broad array of assisted living types and residents, rather than the entire industry of assisted living. For practical and logistical reasons, we chose six facilities in and around the Baltimore–Washington, DC, region. The selection criteria included size, profit status, level of care offered, CS-LTC type, and affiliation (independent or corporate chain). To obtain our study sample, we initially identified and contacted 21 Maryland-based assisted living residences that reflected this diversity. Thirteen of these sites met our criteria and were in operation at the start of the project. From among these, we selected six sites that provided rich diversity in residents' racial/ethnic mix and socioeconomic status, ownership/affiliation, rural and urban location, and size. In the initial phase of the project we met with the executive directors of each assisted living facility to explain the research and gain permission to include their residence in the study. Each of these settings received an honorarium of $2,500 for the benefit of the residents. The administrators used these financial gifts to purchase, for example, a piano, lamps, or a television for a shared living room space.

As noted above, in addition to location and diversity, our criteria for selecting settings included two other primary considerations: level of care and the "model" of assisted living.

LEVEL OF CARE

Licensure for all assisted living homes (both small and large) is based on the levels of care provided to residents who live there. Maryland state regulations define three levels, denoted as 1 (low), 2 (moderate), or 3 (high) and referring to the amount of care provided to each individual.[1] A person who is mentally alert and needs assistance only with bathing and dressing is classified at level

1. Someone classified at level 2 generally needs help with three or four activities of daily living, such as bathing, dressing, walking, and toileting. A person who shows signs of confusion or dementia, has an extensive medication schedule, and needs assistance with bathing, eating, walking, toileting, and dressing is classified at level 3. In Maryland, most facilities (approximately 80 percent) are licensed at level 3; this does not mean that every resident in the setting requires that level of care, merely that the facility is licensed to provide it. There are few homes in Maryland at the lowest level of care because most users of assisted living have developed needs beyond this level of care before seeking such a setting.

An additional level referred to as "3+" permits a facility to provide high-intensity care to an individual who needs sophisticated medical support or hospice, but this designation must be approved by the regulating agency on a case-by-case basis in the form of a Medicaid waiver. This waiver authorizes an assisted living program to continue to care for an individual whose physical or cognitive functioning has changed since admission, as long as the setting can demonstrate that it has the capacity to provide the necessary services without compromising the care of the other residents.

MODELS OF ASSISTED LIVING

As a result of our previous research, we identified three models, or types, of assisted living residences:

- small settings—those that house 15 or fewer residents;

- traditional settings—those built before 1987, often former nursing or congregate homes that have been retrofitted for assisted living; and

- new model settings—those purposefully built after 1987 to address the emergent views and goals of the assisted living movement (Zimmerman, Sloane, and Eckert 2001).

Table 1 summarizes the characteristics of the assisted living facilities participating in the transitions study. As the table shows, assisted living facilities in Maryland vary dramatically in size, a range prompted by the inclusiveness of diverse settings under Maryland's assisted living rules and not characteristic of all states. We studied two examples of each of the three setting types listed above. All of the settings in our sample were for-profit businesses,

TABLE 1 *Characteristics of assisted living facilities studied*

Name	Capacity	Type	Ownership	Setting	Level
Valley Glen Home	6	Small	Owner-operator	Suburban	3
Franciscan House	8	Small	Owner-operator	Suburban	2
Huntington Inn	35	Traditional	Owner-operator	Rural	3
Middlebury Manor	42	Traditional	Family-owned/ operated	Suburban	2
The Chesapeake	100	New-model	Large chain	Suburban	3
Laurel Ridge	112	New-model	Small chain	Suburban	3

whether owned by families or part of corporate chains. As is the case for assisted living facilities at large in Maryland, most were licensed for level 3 care.

Fieldwork

Ethnographic fieldwork (research conducted on site or "in the field") began in April 2002. Fieldwork was initially conducted at the two small assisted living sites, starting with Valley Glen Home and proceeding to Franciscan House. This was followed by interviews and observations at Huntington Inn, a traditional assisted living residence; the Chesapeake, part of a large new-model chain; Middlebury Manor, the second traditional assisted living field site; and finally Laurel Ridge, another new-model assisted living facility. By the summer of 2006, the bulk of the data had been collected. However, there continued to be ongoing contact with administrators and residents to update the research team on relevant and significant transitions, such as relocations or deaths among residents, and also shifts in management, staffing, and ownership.

During the active data collection in the two small assisted living homes, a project ethnographer spent an average of eight hours per week doing field research. In each of the larger traditional and new-model assisted living settings, two project ethnographers conducted fieldwork on average four to five hours per day, two to three days per week for 6–10 months. Time in the field varied, reflecting the various facilities' calendars of events and the availability of interviewees. There were times when the ethnographers arrived at the assisted living facility at breakfast and did not leave until the close of evening activities; other times, an ethnographer would visit for several hours interviewing, observing a committee meeting, gossiping with residents and/or staff members on the front porch, or participating in a craft session. By the end of the period of intensive fieldwork, we had been present at each site various times seven days a week and were therefore able to gain information on life overall inside each residence.

Participant Observation

Participant observation is a key method for conducting ethnographic fieldwork. It involves the on-site observation of the physical and social environment studied and participation in the routines of daily life as they naturally occur in the field. Participant observation relies heavily on insights generated by the ethnographers, based on their knowledge of and experiences in the settings. Extensive field notes, including analytic and expressive commentary, are written at the close of each visit. In our research, these field notes were then compiled, shared with colleagues, coded, and analyzed, as discussed below in the sections on data management and analysis.

One of the ways we gained intimate knowledge of the assisted living settings was to volunteer our time and skills. For example, at Franciscan House we hosted a holiday cookie decorating party, and at the Chesapeake, we helped staff the dining room, refilling coffee cups, serving meals, scraping plates, and clearing tables. Sometimes we ate meals with residents, tasting firsthand the food being served. We also shopped with and for residents, played the piano, walked pets, and offered solace. At Middlebury Manor, we assisted in cleaning out the activities room and recycling a closet full of magazines, and we served desserts and wine and cheese at socials. During our visits to Laurel Ridge we had the opportunity to facilitate a resident's return into the "art world" after her stroke, as well as help with the mundane but appreciated polishing of fingernails. These are but few examples of how we "gave back" to the individuals who supported and contributed to our research efforts.

Ethnographic Interviewing

Another important technique in conducting ethnographic fieldwork is in-depth, open-ended interviewing. Researchers used guides to structure the interview and elicit information from study participants. Asking the same set of broad or open-ended questions of all respondents allowed ethnographers to obtain a core set of data; at the same time, the openness of the questions allowed for extemporaneous responses and follow-ups by the interviewer.

Obtaining data that was respondent-driven freed the ethnographer to explore points of interest specific to one individual and opened up new avenues of thought which were pursued later in the research. Interview guides were flexible and fluid, not fixed or formal. Thus, interview questions were adapted reflexively, with probes to expand on the informants' initial responses.

In each of the six settings, interviews were conducted with multiple informants (another ethnographic term for "interviewee"), including "focal case" residents, as defined below, their family members, selected direct care staff, and administrators. Residents who elected not to participate in the research or who were cognitively unable to give consent were not interviewed. To broaden our knowledge base and to represent the experience of residents with dementia, we interviewed their family members, and observed and noted their interactions in the assisted living residence. Interviews were generally scheduled in advance and tape-recorded. Several residents, however, declined to be taped; therefore, their responses were hand-written by the ethnographer. Several short interviews were conducted informally and compiled in field notes. A number of family members were interviewed over the telephone.

The focus in the interviews was on personal experience, subjective accounts, interpretations, and meaning. Interviews were intended to provide insights into the perspective of each respondent, and they often flowed more like conversations than do the highly structured interviews used in standard survey research. Questions were similar across the groups of residents, families, and staff, but the responses reflected their varied perspectives and positions. For example, the ethnographers asked assisted living residents to describe the series of events leading up to their entry into the setting, and to describe their daily lives, both their pleasures and challenges, now that they had made this transition. Interviews with family members, staff, and administrators provided alternative perspectives on many of the same events and circumstances. All interview guides focused on personal history, transitions, life in assisted living, health, and support. Other sections of the guide addressed topics relevant to a particular respondent category—for example, aspects of work life for direct care staff. Guides for interviewing administrators were tailored toward the specific assisted living facility and addressed such concerns as reactions to new state regulations, increased competition from neighboring assisted living settings, risk management, and creating a dementia care unit.

To supplement the field notes and recorded interviews, we also collected marketing packets, copies of residential contracts, and information on the external environment in which assisted living settings operate, such as materials from policy and regulatory groups.

Extended Focal Case Studies

As part of this data-collection process, ethnographers conducted interviews with more than 150 residents, approximately 100 of whom were identified as "focal cases." Focal cases were selected through purposive sampling, a technique that enables researchers to pursue cases that represent a range of experiences (Patton 1990).

For each focal case, we conducted both formal and informal interviews with the resident and with one or more family members, when family members were available. We also discussed the residents with staff and other professionals, including direct care staff and outside case managers. Copious field notes also contributed to information on these individuals and their daily lives. The following paragraphs provide more detail on the fieldwork and the focal cases described in Chapters 2–7.

The fieldwork for this study began in the spring of 2002 at Valley Glen Home. We made weekly visits for 11 months and then followed up with Rani, mostly by telephone, until spring 2007. Miss Helen was selected as a focal case even though she was incapable of participating in an interview. Instead, we interviewed her daughter and Rani on Miss Helen's behalf, and we saw her at every visit. In addition, she was mentioned in every field note.

We conducted research at Franciscan House from September 2002 through April of 2003 and then followed up with semiannual telephone calls until the spring of 2007. Opal took part in three ethnographic interviews and three supplemental meetings, during which her physical and cognitive status was assessed using standardized tools. She was mentioned in interviews with family members of two other residents and three interviews with Maria, and is described in all field notes. No one in her family was willing to be interviewed for this study.

Fieldwork at Huntington Inn began in December 2002 and continued with weekly visits until November 2003 and periodic visits and telephone calls until spring 2006. Our ethnographers completed four interviews with Karen and one with her son Mark. In addition, the events of Karen's life, including her medical condition, moves into and out of Huntington Inn, and her financial status, were topics of discussion in several formal and informal interviews with Mr. Hill. Karen was mentioned in many interviews with other residents and with staff members and in the majority of field notes.

At the Chesapeake, we collected ethnographic field data between September 2003 and February 2007, with the heaviest concentration acquired in 2004. In addition to participant observation and focused interviewing, two undergraduate interns assisted Dr. Catherine in her quest to bring activities into the dementia care unit by designing and executing art projects involving both her and other residents. The interns also photographed and mapped the setting. In total, there are six interviews relating to Dr. Catherine: one completed by her daughter, four with Dr. Catherine herself, and one assessment protocol. Dr. Catherine is cited in 44 ethnographic field notes and in numerous interviews with residents and staff.

Middlebury Manor fieldwork took place between June 2004 and April 2007, with most fieldwork completed in 2004 and 2005. In total there are nine full-length interviews related to Mrs. Koehler: three with her and six with her daughters. Nearly 50 field notes and four staff interviews include significant mentions of Mrs. Koehler. In total, our research at Middlebury Manor generated nearly 700 pages of field notes and interviews.

We collected ethnographic field data at Laurel Ridge between October 2004 and February 2007, with most of our information collected in 2005 and 2006. One of the residents at Laurel Ridge was an artist; an undergraduate intern photographed the entire collection of her paintings to complete a portfolio for a museum submission. He also visited with residents and took field notes. In total, there are ten interviews related to Mr. Sidney: six with Mr. Sidney himself, one with his wife's great-niece, two with his good friend, Mrs. Perkins, and one with her niece. Mr. Sidney is cited in 23 ethnographic field notes and in interviews with staff members.

For analytic reasons, we considered the focal cases as being nested within a larger-scale "case," the assisted living setting. Participant observation enabled us to identify the distinct and compelling traits of each setting's culture: resident care, business management, social life, rules, and values—all the aspects that make each setting different from others. Thus, we came to describe our design as "case (resident) within case (setting)" research. Chapters 2 through 7 represent the outcome of this analytic approach.

Gaining Trust and Access

Gaining the trust of study participants was necessary to the success of this project. Initial access to the settings and permission to interview individuals were obtained early in the research. However, the quality and accuracy of data collected and the strength of relationships in the assisted living homes were the result of the rapport we established with informants. Residents invited us into their rooms and lives, staff members shared break time, administrators welcomed us to meetings, and families knew firsthand the benefit of our research. Overwhelmingly, participants were receptive and positive. The true test of trust occurred in one assisted living facility where direct care staff shared in confidence their fears of retribution by management should they speak openly with us, which explained why we had difficulty getting interviews with the care aides in that particular setting.

In each setting, we listened as residents spoke glowingly of grandchildren and chastised their children, while staff members confided their frustration with low wages and working weekends. The ethnographers also established rapport with management, hearing their frustrations with retaining good-quality staff, the rising costs of doing business, rude family members, or increasing state requirements. As with all ethnography, it was the informal gate-keeper, a resident or care aide, whose positive opinions of our work helped to open doors. We appreciate the generous invitations to go behind the scenes, introducing us to life "backstage" in assisted living (Goffman 1959).

Data Management and Analysis
Team Approach

As data collection proceeded, field notes were written and interviews recorded and transcribed. This information—in written narrative form—was reviewed by a multidisciplinary team of researchers representing anthropology, sociology, social work, gerontology, and folklore. The research team spent considerable time working as a group, meeting twice a month during the five years of data collection and for another 12 months after. During these bimonthly meetings, the team discussed key similarities and differences among the settings and among the numerous individuals—residents, staff, administrators, and family members—who had shared important details of their lives, both recent and more remote.

Data Storage

Field notes and interview transcripts were stored centrally in a textbase. By the time the field research was complete, more than 15,000 pages of interview transcripts and field notes were generated. To practically manage this amount of narrative data, we entered it into *Atlas.ti* (Muhr 2007), a software program that facilitates qualitative data analysis by enabling researchers to store and retrieve project documents, notes, and specific quotations. *Atlas.ti* allows for text-based searching on particular words or topics and also provides a structure for the input of analytical codes, which essentially constitute the frame of analysis (Charmaz 2006) and render the data meaningful (Lofland et al. 2006). As described below, coding systems permitted retrieval and review of material from this archive of information on transitions to, and lives within, assisted living.

Collaborative Coding Process

A coding framework was developed using the grounded theory approach (Strauss 1987; Strauss and Corbin 1990). Coding is the process of organizing and sorting data, or as Charmaz puts it, the "process of defining what the data are about" (2006, p. 43). Codes are the words used to "organize ideas applied to the items or chunks of data in your field notes or other materials, or to the answers of the questions asked . . . or, more abstractly, the labels we use to classify items of information" (Lofland et al. 2006, p. 200). Coding shapes the framework of analysis, defines what is happening in the field, links data to theory, directs further data gathering, and eventually allows researchers to "sort, synthesize, integrate, and organize large amounts of data" (Charmaz 2006, pp. 45–46). By interacting with and working through the data, researchers capture the meaning of the participants' lived experiences from the insiders' points of view.

In the transitions study, the coding process began early in our fieldwork with initial coding, as the first interviews were returned, and continued through the duration of the project with focused coding identifying pieces of narrative by themes or topics. Interview transcripts were read and reread as researchers worked through the data so that ethnographic material could be categorized and sorted. Field notes and interviews were compared and contrasted until thematic categories emerged to fit the data overall. This process led to the development of a project code book, which, at the conclusion of the study, contained a total of 54 codes.

Rotating two-person coding teams, comprised of investigators, ethnographers, the project coordinator, and graduate research assistants, coded each project document (interview transcripts and field notes) through a collaborative process. Team members first coded the documents separately; coding partners then met to examine their independent analysis and reconcile any differences. Ethnographers did not code their own field notes or interviews. Unresolved questions were discussed during bimonthly project meetings, and codes were reviewed and revised as necessary. New codes (introduced rarely once focused coding commenced) or revised definitions were then entered into *Atlas.ti* for further analysis as the work progressed. Thus, coding allowed the team to identify particular ideas and issues that emerged in the narratives, which could then be retrieved from *Atlas.ti* and analyzed in detail.

Data Mining

Once they were coded, the field notes and interview transcripts were mined for text and quotations relevant to particular topics. For example, narrative sections that had been coded the same way across multiple documents were retrieved and analyzed. Specific codes included *aging in place* (discussions about the accommodations made—or the lack thereof—to allow a resident to decline and/or die in the place of residence or elsewhere), the *meaning of time* (how time is experienced, in finite units, indefinite intervals, or as an ongoing process or temporal dimension), and *maintenance of self* (verbal or behavioral expressions of personal agency, including references to one's own appearance and that of others and cognitive ability, self-medication, mobility, and discussions of personal possessions). Other codes related to quality of care, home operations and management, discussions of money, and the physical and social environment.

The results of structured textbase searches, which could also be restricted to particular assisted living settings or categories of respondents (e.g., residents only), were stored and further refined. Related documents were established as "families" within *Atlas.ti* to facilitate queries on a subset of data, such as all materials from the new-model assisted living facilities. Codes were also combined with other codes or word searches to identify text related to topics, such as autonomy or "settling in" to an assisted living home. To find excerpts related to autonomy, for example, we searched for words such as "independence" and "freedom," and for text coded as *maintenance of self*, as defined above. To find text related to settling in, we searched for variations of the words "settle" and "move," as well as codes for *homelike*, *emotions*, and *transitions*.

Connecting Codes to Narratives

To develop themes and visualize patterns within the data, we connected coded text and quotations to emerging theories or potential explanations for our observations. Memos were generated to record the researchers' thoughts about the data and the project. Sometimes researchers wrote memos while coding the documents or reading through the results of a word or code search. Other times, they wrote memos to record thoughts while reading the documents sequentially. The team used memos and other analytic notes to share and connect ideas across settings and to identify patterns within the data. Then we used them to compare preliminary themes with further observations on site. As the study progressed, for example, we documented in memos the multiple meanings and levels of transitions: personal transitions, peripheral transitions (such as key transitions of children responsible for an older parent's care), setting-specific and corporate changes, and the evolving regulatory environment.

Analytical Processes

On the basis of our observations and the patterns we saw developing, we used *Atlas.ti* individually and in smaller teams to search our coded documents to cross-check and substantiate or dispel our hunches or insights. We conducted structured searches on particular codes or within specified "families" of data related to the topics of interest, and read and reread the narratives in depth. As we prepared for presentations, articles, and the writing of this book, we compared and contrasted experiences within and across focal cases, as well as within individual assisted living settings and across the three categories of assisted living. We connected ideas regarding how particular cases at either the "focal case" level or the assisted living "setting" level informed the issues, dilemmas, and everyday lived experience of assisted living.

Deeper analysis involved identifying themes and testing explanations against data. We identified, for example, a number of themes related to transitions, including our findings that decisions to enter assisted living are likely to be crisis-driven, rather than deliberate consumer choices; that many transitions occur in the same setting without relocation; and that for aging in place to be the right outcome, the fit between the residents' needs and preferences must be balanced with the assisted living setting's ability to meet these needs over time.

Future Research

For more than five years, our research team sat around the bimonthly meeting table, hearing updates from the field, discussing field notes and interviews, and sharing ideas. We used this collective knowledge to analyze themes and patterns we saw develop. Our experiences in the field and our conversations around that meeting table helped us all better understand assisted living settings and the people who live, visit, and work there. The findings presented in this book merely scratch the surface of the knowledge generated by this study. We continue to build on this research, exploring the topics, themes, and insights we have gained.

Productive lines of research emerging from the transitions project include a study of quality in assisted living from the perspective of residents (Morgan, Eckert, and Rubinstein), a study of physician care in assisted living (Schumacher, Eckert, and Zimmerman), a sociocultural study of stigma in senior housing of various types (Eckert, Rubinstein, Morgan, and Zimmerman), the meaning of autonomy (Rubinstein and Frankowski), and policy and practice issues related to medication management (Zimmerman and Carder). Our intention is to pursue these new lines of research to promote a better understanding of life inside assisted living.

Notes

....

Chapter One: Introduction

1. Other possible factors include declining disability rates, widowhood, childlessness among older persons, and certificate-of-need limitations.

2. Oregon was the first state to receive a Home and Community Based Services Waiver from the Centers for Medicare and Medicaid Services. Under that waiver, individuals who qualify for "nursing home level of care" and for the Medicaid financial threshold are eligible to move into an assisted living setting rather than a skilled nursing facility. Individual residents must also apply and are accepted as a recipient after meeting two eligibility standards: (1) the individual must be assessed as needing "nursing home level of care," and (2) the individual must meet the state's Medicaid income criteria. A total of 36 states, including Maryland, have this waiver, and another 24 states have other arrangements to subsidize the cost of assisted living for persons with low incomes (Mollica, Johnson-Lamarche, and O'Keeffe 2005). However, states limit the total number of persons covered by any type of public subsidy for assisted living.

3. The argument for providing private disabled-accessible apartments was based on social science research about the relationship between older individuals and their living environments. Powell Lawton and Lucille Nahemow's (1973) model of environmental press-competence was influential, as was Langer and Rodin's (1976) study of personal control in nursing homes.

4. The American Institute of Architects has a committee called the Design for Aging Knowledge Community that seeks to "foster design innovation and disseminate knowledge necessary to enhance the built environment and quality of life for an aging society" (AIA 2007). The international group organizes workshops on topics such as design for dementia, technology, and community development.

5. The Omnibus Budget and Reconciliation Act of 1987, or OBRA '87.

Chapter Three: Opal at Franciscan House

1. Based on a review of assisted living facilities that are certified to receive Medicaid subsidies as reported on the Maryland Office of Health Care Quality web site (OHCQ 2006).

Chapter Four: Karen at Huntington Inn

1. As part of their application to the Centers for Medicare and Medicaid Services for a 1915c waiver, states must specify a limit on the number of individuals who may receive specified services. The number limits are referred to as "slots" (LeBlanc, Tonner, and Harrington 2000).

Chapter Five: Mrs. Koehler at Middlebury Manor

1. Before Congress enacted provisions to the Social Security Act, community-dwelling spouses of nursing home patients were at risk of becoming impoverished by the cost of their partner's nursing home care. The 1988 provision, known as "spousal impoverishment," helps prevent community spouses from depleting their financial resources in order to pay for their partner's care.

Chapter Nine: Aging in Places

1. Some assisted living facilities (half of those in our study) charge a "community fee," a one-time charge at the time when the resident moves in or at a specified time thereafter (e.g., 30 days). As noted in Chapter 5, the community fee is a one-time charge to cover costs for maintenance and upkeep of the building. This charge ranged from $1,500 to several thousands of dollars in the residences in our study.

Chapter Ten: The Reality and the Promise of Assisted Living

1. Assisted living organizations include the National Alliance to Improve Assisted Living Care, which is composed of 15 elder care, elder law, and senior advocacy groups promoting stronger consumer protections for assisted living residents, and the Center for Excellence in Assisted Living, which is a clearinghouse for research, state regulations, and licensing concerning assisted living, intended to promote high-quality assisted living, best practices, and policy. Other long-term care organizations include the National Commission for Quality Long-Term Care, which has focused on six broad areas needing change: the culture of long-term care itself, the empowerment of individuals and families, the assisted living workforce, technology, regulation, and finance.

1. The Maryland regulations [2 Maryland Health-General 19-1801. 310. 07.14.10J (1)–(7)] outline seven conditions under which an assisted living program may not admit an individual. Services may not be provided if, at the time of initial assessment, the individual requires (1) more than intermittent nursing care; (2) treatment of stage 3 or stage 4 skin ulcers; (3) ventilator services; (4) skilled monitoring, testing, and aggressive adjustment of medications and treatments where there is the presence of, or risk for, a fluctuating acute condition; (5) monitoring of a chronic medical condition that is not controllable through readily available medications and treatments; (6) treatment for an active reportable communicable disease; or (7) treatment for a disease or condition which requires more than contact isolation.

References

AIA (American Institute of Architects). 2007. *Design for Aging*. Knowledge Community. www.aia.org.

ALW (Assisted Living Workgroup). 2003. *Assuring quality in assisted living: Guidelines for federal and state policy, state regulations, and operations*. A report to the U.S. Senate Special Committee on Aging from the Assisted Living Workgroup. Washington, DC: ALW.

Assisted Living Federation of America. 2007. *ALFA Web Site*.www.alfa.org.

Ball, M. M., M. M. Perkins, F. J. Whittington, B. Connell, and C. Hollingsworth. 2004. Managing decline in assisted living: The key to aging in place. *Journal of Gerontology: Social Sciences* 59(4): S202–12.

Bernard, S., S. Zimmerman, and J. K. Eckert. 2001. Aging-in-place. In *Assisted living: Needs, practices, and policies in residential care for the elderly*, ed. S. Zimmerman, P. D. Sloane, and J. K. Eckert. Baltimore: Johns Hopkins University Press.

Bruce, P. A. 2006. The ascendancy of assisted living: The case for federal regulation. *Elder Law Journal* 14(1): 61–89.

Calkins, M. 2001. The physical and social environment of the person with Alzheimer's disease. *Aging and Mental Health* 5(1S): S74–78.

Carder, P. C. 2002a. The social world of assisted living. *Journal of Aging Studies* 16: 1–18.

———. 2002b. Promoting independence: An analysis of assisted living facility marketing materials. *Research on Aging* 24: 106–23.

Carder, P. C., and M. Hernandez. 2004. Consumer discourse in assisted living. *Journal of Gerontology: Social Sciences* 59B: S58–67.

Carder, P. C., L. M. Morgan, and J. K. Eckert. 2008. The fragile future of small board-and-care homes. In *The assisted living residence: A vision for the future*, ed. S. Golant and J. Hyde. Baltimore: Johns Hopkins University Press.

Carlson, E. 2005. *Critical issues in assisted living: Who's in, who's out, and who's providing the care?* Washington, DC: National Senior Citizens Law Center.

CBS Evening News. 2006. Assisted living, erratic regulation: With no federal regulation and limited state laws, negligence cases are growing, November 13. www.cbsnews.com/stories/2006/11/13/cbsnews_investigates/main2177892.shtml.

Chapin, R., and D. Dobbs-Kepper. 2001. Aging-in-place in assisted living: Philosophy versus policy. *The Gerontologist* 41: 43–50.

Charmaz, K. 2006. *Constructing grounded theory.* Thousand Oaks, CA: Sage Publications.

Consumer Reports. 2005. CR investigates assisted living: How much assistance can you really count on? *Consumer Reports* 70(7): 28.

Day, K., D. Carreon, and C. Stump. 2000. Therapeutic design of environments for people with dementia: A review of the empirical research. *The Gerontologist* 40(4): 397–416.

Dobkin, L. 1989. *The board and care system: A regulatory jungle.* Washington, DC: AARP.

Eckert, J. K., L. A. Morgan, and N. Swamy. 2004. Preferences for receipt of care among community-dwelling adults. *Journal of Aging and Social Policy* 16(2): 49–66.

Ekerdt, D. J., J. F. Sergeant, M. Dingel, and M. E. Bowen. 2004. Household disbandment in later life. *Journal of Gerontology: Social Sciences* 59B: S265–73.

Frank, J. B. 2002. *The paradox of aging in place in assisted living.* Westport, CT: Bergin & Garvey.

GAO (U.S. General Accounting Office). 1999. *Assisted living: Quality-of-care and consumer protection issues in four states.* GAO/HEHS-99-27. Washington, DC: GAO.

Goffman, E. R. 1959. *The presentation of self in everyday life.* New York: Anchor Books.

Golant, S. 2005/06. Supportive housing for frail, low-income older adults: Identifying need and allocating resources. *Generations* 29(4): 37–43.

———. 2008. The future of assisted living residences: A response to uncertainty. Chap. 1 in *The assisted living residence: A vision for the future*, ed. S. Golant and J. Hyde. Baltimore: Johns Hopkins University Press.

Hawes, C., C. D. Phillips, and M. Rose. 2000. *High-service or high-privacy assisted living facilities: Their residents and staff; Results from a national survey.* Office of the Assistant Secretary for Planning and Evaluation (ASPE) of the U.S. Department of Health and Human Services and Texas A&M University System Health Science Center. Washington, DC.

Hawes, C., J. Wildfire, V. Mor, V. Wilcox, D. Spore, V. Iannacchione, et al. 1995. *A description of board and care facilities, operators, and residents.* Research Triangle Park, NC: Research Triangle Institute, Program on Aging and Long-Term Care, Health and Social Policy Division.

Hawes, C., C. D. Phillips, M. Rose, S. Holan, and M. Sherman. 2003. A national survey of assisted living facilities. *The Gerontologist* 43(6): 875–82.

Justice, D., and A. Heestand. 2003. Promising practices in long-term-care systems reform: Oregon's HCBS System. Washington, DC: Medstat.

Kane, R. A., and K. B. Wilson. 2001. Assisted living at the crossroads: Principles for its future. Discussion paper prepared for Summit on Regulating Assisted Living, September, 2001. Portland, OR: Jessie F. Richardson Foundation.

Kinnaman, J. 1949. The nursing home: A medical care facility. *American Journal of Public Health Nations Health* 39: 1099–1105.

Langer, E., and J. Rodin. 1976. The effects of choice and enhanced personal responsibility for the aged. *Journal of Personality and Social Psychology* 34: 191–98.

Lawton, M. 1981. Alternative housing. *Journal of Gerontological Social Work* 3(3): 61–80.

Lawton, M. P., and L. Nahemow. 1973. Ecology and the aging process. In *Psychology of adult development and aging,* ed. C. Eisdorfer and M. P. Lawton. Washington, DC: American Psychological Association.

LeBlanc, A. J., M. C. Tonner, and C. Harrington. 2000. Medicaid 1915 (c) home and community-based services waivers across the states. *Health Care Financing Review* 22(2): 159–74.

Lee, G. R., C. W. Peek, and R. T. Cowart. 1998. Race difference in filial responsibility: Expectations among older adults. *Journal of Marriage and the Family* 60: 404–12.

Levey, S., and R. Amidon. 1967. The evolution of extended care facilities. *Nursing Homes,* August, pp. 14–19.

Lofland, J., D. Snow, L. Anderson, and L. H. Lofland. 2006. *Analyzing social settings.* Belmont, CA: Wadsworth/Thomson Learning.

Matthews, S. 2002. *Sisters and brothers / daughters and sons: Meeting the needs of old parents.* Bloomington, IN: Unlimited Publishing.

Mead, L. C., J. K. Eckert, S. Zimmerman, and J. G. Schumacher. 2005. Sociocultural aspects of transitions from assisted living for residents with dementia. *The Gerontologist* 45: 115–23.

Mendelson, M. A. 1974. *Tender loving greed.* New York: Vintage Books.

MetLife. 2005. *The MetLife market survey of assisted living costs.* Westport, CT: MetLife Mature Market Institute.

Mollica, R. L., H. Johnson-Lamarche, and Janet O'Keeffe. 2005. *State residential care and assisted living policy, 2004.* March 31, 2005. www.aspe.hhs.gov/daltcp/reports/04alcom.htm.

Morgan, L. A., J. K. Eckert, and S. L. Lyon. 1995. *Small board-and-care homes: Residential care in transition.* Baltimore: Johns Hopkins University Press.

Morgan, L. A., A. L. Gruber-Baldini, and J. Magaziner. 2001. Resident characteristics. In *Assisted living: Needs, practices, and policies in residential care for the elderly,* ed. S. Zimmerman, P. D. Sloane, and J. K. Eckert. Baltimore: Johns Hopkins University Press.

Muhr, T. 2007. *Atlas.ti* version 5.2.11. Berlin: Scientific Software Development.

NCAL (National Center for Assisted Living). 2007. *2006 Overview of assisted living.* Washington, DC: NCAL.

NCHS (National Center for Health Statistics). 2007. National home and hospice care data description. January 11. www.cdc.gov/nchs/about/major/nhhcsd/nhhcsdes.htm.

NORC Public Policy. 2007. National Public Policy Outlook for NORC Supportive Services. *NORCs: An Aging-in-Place Retirement Initiative.* www.norcs.com/page.html?ArticleID=138431.

OHCQ (Maryland Office of Health Care Quality). 2005. *Maryland's assisted living program 2005 evaluation: Final report and regulations.* January 2006. www.dhmh.state.md.us/ohcq/alforum/2005_alp_rpt.pdf.

———. 2006. *OHCQ Web site.* www.dhmh.state.md.us/ohcq.

O'Keeffe, J., and J. M. Wiener. 2004. Public funding for long-term care services for older people in residential care settings. *Journal of Housing for the Elderly* 18(3/4): 51–79.

Pastalan, L. 1990. *Aging in place: The role of housing and social support.* New York: Haworth Press.

Patton, M. 1990. *Qualitative evaluation and research methods.* Newbury Park, CA: Sage Publications.

Phillips, C. D., Y. Munoz, M. Sherman, M. Rose, W. Spector, and C. Hawes. 2003. Effects of facility characteristics on departures from assisted living: Results from a national study. *The Gerontologist* 43(5): 690–96.

Prisuta, R., L. Barrett, and E. L. Evans. 2006. *Aging, migration, and local communities: The views of 60+ residents and community leaders; An executive summary.* Washington, DC: AARP.

Pynoos, J., P. H. Feldman, and J. Ahrens., eds. 2004. *Linking housing and services for older adults: Obstacles, options, and opportunities.* Binghamton, NY: Haworth Press.

Redfoot, D. 2005. Assisted living and the changing face of aging: Managing the monster. Paper presented at the American Society on Aging annual meeting, Philadelphia.

Regnier, V. 1997. *Assisted living housing for the elderly: Design innovations from the United States and Europe.* New York: Wiley.

Rosenblatt, A., Q. M. Samus, C. D. Steele, A. S. Baker, M. G. Harper, J. Brandt, et al. 2004. The Maryland assisted living study: Prevalence, recognition, and treatment of dementia and other psychiatric disorders in the assisted living population of central Maryland. *Journal of the American Geriatric Society* 52: 1618–25.

Rubinstein, R. L. 1989. The home environments of older people: A description of the psychosocial processes linking person to place. *Journal of Gerontology: Social Sciences* 44: S45–53.

San Antonio, P. M., and R. L. Rubinstein. 2004. Long-term care planning as a cultural system. *Journal of Aging and Social Policy* 16(2): 35–48.

Sarton, M. 1982. *As we are now.* New York: Norton.

Savishinsky, J. S. 2003. "Bread and butter" issues: Food, conflict, and control in a nursing home. In *Gray areas: Ethnographic encounters with nursing home culture,* ed. P. B. Stafford, pp. 103–20. Santa Fe, NM: School of American Research Press.

Schneider, D. M. 1984. *A critique of the study of kinship.* Ann Arbor: University of Michigan Press.

SDSD (Senior and Disabled Service Division). 1989. Assisted living: A social model approach to services. Unpublished report available from Oregon Seniors and Persons with Disabilities, Department of Health and Human Services, 500 Summer St., NE, Salem, OR 97310.

Shalala, D. 1993. Reader feedback. *Assisted Living Today* 1(1): 5.

Shapiro, J. P. 2001. Growing old in a good home. *U.S. News and World Report Health Quarterly* 130(2): 56–61.

Sherman, S. R., and E. S. Newman. 1988. *Foster families for adults: A community alternative in LTC.* New York: Columbia University Press.

Starr, P. 1982. *The social transformation of American medicine.* New York: Basic Books.

Stone, R. 2000. *Long-term care for the elderly with disabilities: Current policy, emerging trends, and implications for the twenty-first century.* New York: Milbank Memorial Fund.

Strauss, A. 1987. *Qualitative analysis for social scientists.* New York: Cambridge University Press.

Strauss, A., and J. Corbin. 1990. *The basics of qualitative research: Grounded theory procedures and techniques.* Newbury Park, CA: Sage Publications.

Thomas, W. H. 2001. *The Eden alternative handbook: The art of building human habitats.* Sherburne, NY: Summer Hill Company.

———. 2006. *What are old people for? How elders will save the world.* Acton, MA: VanderWyk & Burnham.

Vladeck, B. 1980. *Unloving care: The nursing home tragedy.* New York: Basic Books.

Weiner, A., and J. L. Ronch, eds. 2003. *Culture change in long term care.* Binghamton, NY: Haworth Press.

Wilson, K. B. 1990. Assisted living: The merger of housing and long term care services. *Long Term Care Advances* 1: 1–8.

———. 2007. A brief history of the evolution of assisted living in the United States from 1979–2003: Key concepts to anchor a research agenda. *The Gerontologist* 47: 8–22.

Yankelovich, D. 1990. *Long-term care in America: Public attitudes and possible solutions.* Washington, DC: AARP.

Yeoman, B., and D. Peebles. 2006. Rethinking the commune. *AARP: The Magazine.* Washington, DC: AARP.

Zimmerman, S., P. D. Sloane, and J. K. Eckert, eds. 2001. *Assisted living: Needs, practices, and policies in residential care for the elderly.* Baltimore: Johns Hopkins University Press.

Zimmerman, S., A. L. Gruber-Baldini, P. D. Sloane, J. K. Eckert, J. R. Hebel, L. A. Morgan, et al. 2003. Assisted living and nursing homes: Apples and oranges? *The Gerontologist* 43: 101–17.

Zimmerman, S., P. D. Sloane, C. S. Williams, P. S. Reed, J. S. Preisser, J. K. Eckert, et al. 2005a. Dementia care and quality of life in assisted living and nursing homes. *The Gerontologist* 45 (Special Issue 1): 133–46.

Zimmerman, S., P. D. Sloane, J. K. Eckert, A. L. Gruber-Baldini, L. A. Morgan, J. R. Hebel, et al. 2005b. How good is assisted living? Findings and implications from an outcomes study. *Journal of Gerontology: Social Sciences* 60B: S195–204.

Zinn, L. 1999. A good look back over our shoulders. *Nursing Homes/Long-term Care Management,* December, pp. 20–54.

Index

Page numbers in italics indicate table.

board and care, 8, 11, 215
business issues: at Franciscan House, 46–49; overview of, 203–5. *See also* cost issues

caregiving: sibling relationships and, 81–82; stresses of, 91
case manager, involvement of: at Huntington Inn, 67; in search for facility, 18–19; at Valley Glen Home, 25–26
Catherine, Dr. (resident): activities of, 108–9; alcohol consumption by, 100, 118–19; description of, 98–99, 103; dog of, 98, 102, 117–18; health of, 116; on independence, 113–14; redecoration of suite of, 101; Smith and, 102–3, 111–12; transition to dementia care unit by, 117–19
Center for Medicare and Medicaid Services, 201, 229n2
challenges of assisted living: advocacy and policy-oriented groups and, 211; affordability, 73, 209–10; for consumers, 210–11; dynamic environment, 212; dynamic policy and regulatory context, 205–6; shifting consumer preferences and options, 209; success of aging in place, 207; sustaining good-quality workforce, 208–9
change, categories of: finances, 65–67; health, 67–71, 187; overview of, 186–87; public policies, 72–73; in residents, 71–72; rules, 73–74
change, social interpretation of, 187–89
Chesapeake: activities at, 102, 108–9; church subsidy at, 105; dementia unit at, 107; description of, 78; employees, 109–10; exterior of, 104–5; family as primary consumer for, 173–74, 179–80; fieldwork at, 222; food at, 153–54; independence at, 113–15, 119–20; interior of, 106–8; level of care at, 105–6; lifestyle change and, 120–21; marketing of, 178; meal times at, 110–11; medication policy at, 114–15, 121; participant observation at, 103–4; reputation of, 110; residents, 105–6, 121–23, 157; risk agreements at, 115–16; rules of, 109; smokers

and, 102, 114; social relations at, 111–13; social space of, 105–6
choice, constraints on: at Chesapeake, 115–16, 119–20; at Franciscan House, 40–41; health outcomes and, 118–19, 161–62; at Laurel Ridge, 141–42; variations in, by operator, 150. *See also* autonomy, boundaries of
church, relationship of, with Chesapeake, 105
Clare (assistant director): on activity level, 108; as administrator, 123; on aging in place, 167; on discharging residents, 122; on fit, 122–23; on "home," 100–101; on residents appropriate for facility, 105–6; on risk agreements, 115; on transition to dementia unit, 117, 119
Clinton, Mrs. (resident), 139, 140, 146
co-housing communities, 209
Collaborative Studies of Long-Term Care (CS-LTC) typology, 214
community connections, 64–65, 84–85
community fee, 87, 140, 176
competition in market, 136
confidentiality issues, 215
consumer: challenges for, 210–11; definition of, 173, 179–80
consumer-driven model of care: cost issues and, 73; heterogeneity of facilities and, 196–97; limitations on, 172–74; reticence to move and, 146–47; shifting preferences and options in, 209
Consumer Reports investigation, 3
continuing care retirement community, 77
core realities: business matters, 203–5; crisis decision making, 199–200; dynamic lives within dynamic environments, 198–99; fit matters, 203; heterogeneity, 195–98; negotiation of aging in place, 200; people matter, 202–3; place matters, 201–2
cost issues: as criteria for selection of facility, 175–76; departures and, 190–91; at Laurel Ridge, 132–33, 136; for low- to moderate-income seniors, 73,